MATERNAL HEALTH; PREGNANCY, MORBIDITY, and MORTALITY

A Traumatic Experience

ELEANORE CHILLIS

iUniverse books may be ordered through booksellers or by contacting:

iUniverse
1663 Liberty Drive
Bloomington, IN 47403
www.iuniverse.com
844-349-9409

Because of the dynamic nature of the Internet, any web addresses or links contained in this book may have changed since publication and may no longer be valid. The views expressed in this work are solely those of the author and do not necessarily reflect the views of the publisher, and the publisher hereby disclaims any responsibility for them.

Any people depicted in stock imagery provided by Getty Images are models, and such images are being used for illustrative purposes only. Certain stock imagery © Getty Images.

Cover Credit to Olivia Brown
Image Credit to Yusef Morris

ISBN: 978-1-6632-6152-6 (sc)
ISBN: 978-1-6632-6151-9 (e)

Library of Congress Control Number: 2024906366

Print information available on the last page.

iUniverse rev. date: 04/24/2024

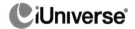

"Take charge and be in charge". — Eleanore Chillis

MATERNAL HEALTH; PREGNANCY, MORBIDITY and MORTALITY

WORD DEFINITIONS:

MORBIDITY: refers to an illness or disease; having a disease or a symptom of disease, or to the amount of disease within a population. Also refers to medical problems caused by treatment.
(mor-BIH-dih-tee)

MORTALITY: refers to death; subject to dying, deaths in large amounts, a measurement of deaths due to a certain area; # of deaths to disease divided by the total population.
(mor-tal-i-ty)

Note: not to be confused with morality

MORALITY: pertaining to morals or manners
(mor-ral-i-ty)

MEDICAL WORD ABBREVIATIONS

abd	abdomen
Abn	abnormal
adm	admission
AFI	Amniotic fluid index
AFP	alpha fetaprotein
AGA	Appropriate for gestational age
atl.	alternate, alternating
UTI	urinary tract infection
AMA	Against Medical Advice
AMB	ambulatory
AMI	Acute Myocardial Infarction
amnio	amniocentesis
bil.	bilateral
BP	blood pressure
c/o	Complaining of patient
C/S	Cesarean section
C/W	consistent with
CBR	complete bed rest
cl	clear
CNA	certified nurses aid
CRNA	Certified Registered Nurse Anesthetist
CST	Contraction stimulation test
D.O.S.	Day of surgery
D.R.	Delivery ROOM
d/c-dc	discontinue
DAT	Diet as tolerated
DTR	Deep tendon reflexes
DVT	Deep venous thrombosis
decr	decrease or diminish

DFA	diet for age
diag	diagnosis
disp	dispense
dang	drainage
EBL	Estimate blood loss
EDC	Estimated date of conception
FACH	forceps after coming head
FM	fetal movement
FMC	Family Maternity Center
FH	family history
fdg	feeding
fl.	fluid
Fl. dr.	fluid dram
fl. oz.	Fluid ounce
FOB	
f.o.b.	foot of bed
GA	gestational assessment
HBP	High Blood Pressure
HPI	history of present illness
HPTN	hypertension
hr,h	hour
hi	history
I.V.	intravenous
id.	the same
IFM	internal fetal monitorl
IMV	inferior Myocardial Infarction
incr	increase
inj	injection
IUGR	intra-uterine pressure catheter
IVAC	intra-venous infusion pump
lb.	pound
L.E.	Lupus Erythematosis
L/D	Labor & Delivery
LA	left arm
LBW	low blood weight
LDR	Labor Delivery
LDRP	Labor Delivery
lg.	large

LMP	Last menstrual period
Lt. L	Left leg
MUM	Mom/Baby Unit
Mg	Magnesium
MH	medical history
NICU	Neonatal Intensive Care Unit
NNP	Neonatal Nurse Practitioner
N	normal
N/C	no complaints
N/A	Nurse Aide
NB	New Born
OB	Obstetrics
OOB	out of bed
OR	Operating Room
OSA	Obstructive sleep apnea
PDN	Private Duty Nurse
PH	past history
PIH	pregnancy induced hypertension
PMH	point medical history
POD	Post Op Day
PPTL	Postpartum tubal ligation
prep	prepare for
PRN	as necessary
P.R.O.M.	partial range of motion
RHD	rheumatoid arthritis fact
RN	Registered Nurse
Rpt	repeat
RR	Recovery Room
RTC	return to clinic
Rt.L	right leg
SAA	same as above
SIDS	Sudden Infant Death Syndrome
Surg.	Surgery
UO	urine output
UTI	urinary tract infection
WHC	Women's Health Clinic

MEDICAL REPORT AND RECORD IMAGE INSERTS LISTED

Medical Report, Record and Photo Image Listed - ix
Dedication - xii (p1)
Constituents - xiv (f2)

Ch 2 - (p3)
Ch 2 - (p4)

Ch 4 - (f5): Discharged Instruction - (10/21/96), 11:45 a.m.

Ch 5 - (f6), (f7), (f8), (f9), (f10), (f11), (f12), (f13): 24 Hour Urine Specimens Collection - (2/24/97 - 2/26/97)
Obstetric Admitting Record - (2/27/97)
Medical History Summary
Admission Progress Note 1
Admission Progress Note 2
Continuation Consultation Sheet 1
Continuation Consultation Sheet 2
Patient Suspicious

Ch 6 - (f14), (f15): Medication Administration Record - 14 Day Schedule Medication - (2/27/97 - 3/8/97)
Parenteral Fluid Record - (3/7/97)

Ch 7 - (f16-a), (f16), (f17): Amniocentesis Tube/Needles - (3/4/97)
Progress Report Afternoon Contractions - (3/4/97)
Progress Report Continued

Ch 10 - (f18), (f19), (f20), (f21), (f22), (f23), (f24), (f25), (f26), (f27): Intra-Operative Care Plan - (3/8/97)
Operative Report - (3/8/97, 3/10/97)
Operative Continued

Labor & Delivery Summary - (3/8/97)
Surgery Record - (3/8/97)
Surgery Pathology Consultation - (3/8/97)
Surgery Pathology Consultation Continued - (3/10/97)
Episodes Following Surgery - (3/8/97)
Episodes Continued

Ch 10 - Continued: (p28), (p29), (p30), (p31), f32), (f33): Preoperative Anesthesia
Evaluation Notes - (3/7/97)
Anesthesia Record & Pre-Anesthesia Medication - (3/8/97)
Preoperative Anesthesia Evaluation Notes - (3/7/97)
Anesthesia Record Continued

Ch 11 - (f34), (f35): Pain Management Flow Sheet - (3/8/97)
Pain Management Flow Sheet Continued - (3/8/97)

Ch 14 - (p36-a&36-b), (p37), (p38), (p39): Wheelchair Mishap - (3/10/97)

Ch 16 - (f40), (f41), (f42), (p43), (p44-a&p44-b), (p45-a&p45-b), (p46): Discharged
Summary - (3/12/97)
Obstetrical and Short-Stay GYN Discharge Summary - (3/12/97)

MATERNAL HEALTH; PREGNANCY, MORBIDITY, and MORTALITY

A Traumatic Experience

BY ELEANORE CHILLIS

A retired Erie County public servant who has accumulated a wealth of experience and knowledge in public and environmental health services, health and wellness, and gives credence to pregnancy trauma and more!

DEDICATION

This book is dedicated to my beloved mother (Hazel) who endured the birth of carrying ten healthy babies to full term. (Although, there were numerous complications that she endured to her personally with the delivering of her last birth and complained often about such female issues until she passed in 2021). I loved her strength and disciplinary ways and took it to heart. To Dr. Uzo Ihenko and son Kelechi, your time and commitment has been unparalleled, trusted, and worthy of all others.

Mom and sister Karin below at the time of Kelechi's birth and all the trauma that pursued.

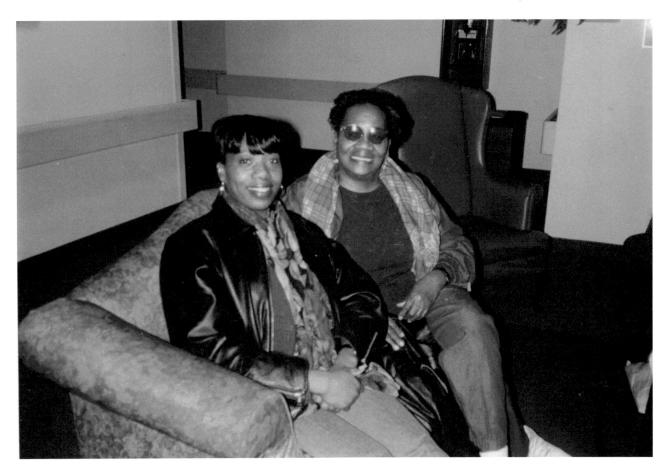

MISSION STATEMENT

Arming women with the tools to avoid maternal health; pregnancy morbidity, and mortality issues through education and demanding they be heard when complaining of subjective pain and symptons.

ACKNOWLEDGEMENTS

Thank you mom and thank you dad for giving your 10 children a two parent home. And Grandmother Clara (Ball) Wright who lived to be 100 years old.

My parents, Mr. and Mrs. Ulysses and Hazel Chillis both originated from the south. My mother passed in 2021 (She was the daughter of Arthur Wright & Clara Wright of Wrightsville, Ga.). Mr. Chillis passed in 2016, he was the epitome of a strong fatherly figure in the household and the son of Gainer Chillis & Hattie Linder of Dublin, Ga.

My roots are from a plantation called Wrightsville, Georgia (the crossing where Sherman Walker marched on to the sea after the American 1861-1865, Civil War) and pioneered in 1866 by John B. Wright, the fifth richest slave owner in the south during slavery. Because my extended family are still living in Wrightsville, in 1988, 1994 and 1996, I personally took the liberty to meet with his great, great granddaughter and visited the gated burial site of our ancestors on the nearby property. Directly across the road from the Phillips Wright family House, a gated cemetery for JBW's family with some black people buried outside of the gate. Down the road in the back of the field is where most of my ancestors are buried.

My parents were the historic 2nd wave of the migrants moving up north. They moved to Buffalo, N.Y. with my fathers, brothers and sisters all from Dublin, Ga. They all belonged to the family Church, New Hope COGIC, 285 Masten Ave. founded by my Uncle Ureese Chillis (the late Superintendent) in 1963-2004. Pastor Chillis started the media campaign, *"Have you prayed about it?"* Opened for all to join. And, *"Ask the Pastor."* Summertimes were spent in Bible Study, studying under the tutelage of Uncle Ureese and his brothers and sisters.

Although COGIC Church was a family Church where we gathered for holidays and sometimes Sunday school. Oftentimes, my brothers and sisters and I would attend other nearby community churches in walking distance. The Shiloh Baptist, 15 Pine St. and Durham Memorial A.M.E. Zion Church, 200 E. Eagle St. as well.

Grandmother Clara remained loyal to Wrightsville where she cooked for the Smith family her whole life. She remained the matriarch for generations up until her passing in 1996. She was such a strong lady, who had never been sickly or hospitalized in her life. She also was known to have taken a daily swig of turpentine for good measures.

NOTE TO BUFFALO CONSTITUENTS

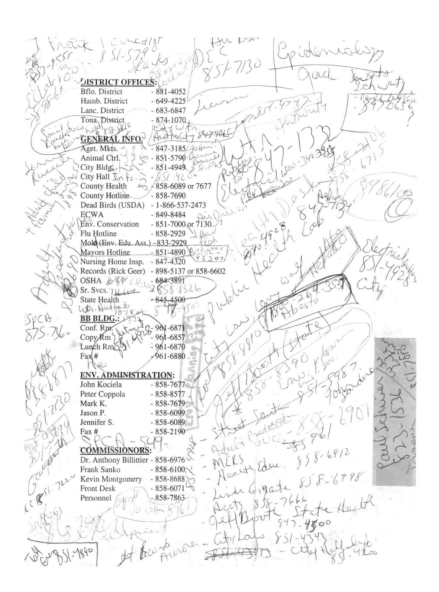

When you called in a complaint, I heard you and it was my joyous honor to have given you a listening ear, whether it was for housing, landlords, lead poisoning, food related illness, restaurant violations or a Freedom Of Information Law (FOIL) request. I was the voice on the other end of the phone and wrote countless complaints one after the other and was very happy to have assisted you. Why? Because I matter and you mattered too! Public Health works relentlessly to protect and keep the public from harm. Therefore, never be intimidated or take no for an answer.

CONTENTS

FOREWORD: 1 xvii

FOREWORD: 2 xix

INTRODUCTION xx

CHAPTER 1   HOW WE MET: 1993 1

CHAPTER 2   PLANNED PREGNANCY: 1996 2

CHAPTER 3   CONFIRMED PREGNANCY AND DUE DATES: 7/24/1996 & 5/2/1997 5

CHAPTER 4   PRENATAL VISITS: 1996 - 2/24/1997 6

CHAPTER 5   HOSPITAL ADMISSION: 2/27/1997 9

CHAPTER 6   BETAMETHASONE SHOT: (1ST DOSE) 2/28/1997 19

CHAPTER 7   AMNIOCENTESIS: 3/4/1997 23

CHAPTER 8   THE NIGHT BEFORE THE EPIDURAL: 3/7/1997 27

CHAPTER 9   BETAMETHASONE SHOT (2ND DOSE): 3/7/1997 28

CHAPTER 10   MAGNESIUM SULFATE: 3/7/1997 - 3/9/1997 29

CHAPTER 11   ANESTHESIOLOGISTS: 3/8/1997 47

CHAPTER 12   ANESTHESIA: 3/8/1997 51

CHAPTER 13   JOURNEY THROUGH THE TUNNEL: 3/8/1997 52

CHAPTER 14   WHEELCHAIR MISHAP: 3/10/1997 54

CHAPTER 15   FIBROIDS: 3/10/1997 60

CHAPTER 16   SENT HOME WITHOUT MEDS: 3/12/1997 62

CHAPTER 17   LEARNING TO WALK AGAIN: 3/15/1997 - 6/15/1997 71

CHAPTER 18   INFANT MORBIDITY, MORTALITY OR SIDS: 4/6/1997 - 4/1998 (VOLUME #2) 73

SPECIAL THANKS...75

IN REMEMBRANCE OF 77

OPERATIVE REPORT MEDICAL TERMS 78

OPERATIVE REPORT MEDICAL TERMS & DEFINITIONS...79

OPERATIVE REPORT MEDICAL TERMS & PROCEDURES DURING C-SECTION 82

PREGNANCY RELATED TERMS 84

LINKS 92

REFERENCES 99

GLOSSARY A - Z 106

STORY LINKS...110

RELATED STORY LINKS..111

OBTAINING MEDICAL RECORDS, REPORT AND INCIDENT REPORTS 130

FILING A COMPLAINT..133

PATIENT SAFETY...134

PATIENT NON-COMPLIANCE— A POWERFUL LEGAL DEFENSE 142

HOW CAN I COMPLAIN ABOUT POOR MEDICAL CARE I RECEIVED IN A HOSPITAL?............145

ADDENDUM..147

AUTHOR'S BIO 148

INDEX 149

FOREWORD: 1

Twenty-six years ago, the author Ms. Eleanore Chillis had her one and only child. During these periods of pregnancy, birth, and child development she and the baby were faced with many hospital and doctor missed and oversight diagnoses that nearly posed health challenges or death to both mother and child.

It is these hospital and real life experiences through pregnancy and child rearing that uniquely position and give credence to this book and to the author. As a result, the author has determined to share her real-life experiences and knowledge to bring awareness and to educate other women, especially expectant mothers with their respective husbands or significant other, on the challenges women face during pregnancies and childbirth. The request to write a foreword on this piece of work was very delightful and honorable. My name is Dr. Uzo Ihenko, president and CEO of Uzo 1 International, Ltd., an international corporation headquartered in Buffalo, New York. I attended the State University of New York at Buffalo where I obtained a Ph.D in urban geography with specialization in urban and regional analysis.

Thirty years ago, I became personally acquainted with Ms. Chillis. Over the years, our friendship and relationship grew as we became the family through which our son was born. Throughout these periods whereby we lived as family, I have come to know Ms. Chillis as a very loving and caring person. She loves her family so much and cherished her son so dearly. This caring attribute has now extended to others in the community. She has devoted her life to learning and acquiring even more knowledge on life's safety measures to serve our community. College educated, she has worked in varied industries at various capacities that include Public and Environmental Health Services.

Contrarily, as it may seem, the author was not alone in her pregnancy and childbirth experience. Although I did not carry the baby for seven months nor did I give birth to a baby, I was by her side throughout the ordeal. I was up when she was up and at the hospital whenever she had to go. Hence, one can argue that I too had faced some level of childbirth trauma. Equally revealing is the courage and tenacity Ms. Chillis had in keeping her new baby son alive. She has low tolerance for doctors who provide wrong diagnostics and could not explain any health condition the baby was experiencing. She never ceased to obtain a second opinion and never settled with any explanation that did not make any sense to her about the son's health. At times, I used to be disappointed by her tenacity but later realized that her courage and tenacity was in part what kept the baby alive.

Similarly, Ms. Chillis has now taken her energy to saving others through her book. The author has grounded knowledge and deep real-life experience to the subject matter for which is detailed in her book.

In volume one, her book is designed to tell her traumatic story and "*arming women with the tools to avoid maternal health; pregnancy morbidity, and mortality issues through education and demanding they be heard while complaining of subjective pain and systems, getting the necessary unbiased care to help improve their outcomes, and utilizing medical records and report findings to help women and expectant mothers make life-informed decisions.*" Furthermore, her next book on "INFANT MORBIDITY, MORTALITY or SIDS" Volume two speaks on how to look after and protect the newborn baby.

I, therefore, am deeply appreciative and admire the level of work the author has put forward to the readers. I am also proud and delighted to have contributed through writing the foreword for the book. Personally, I would strongly recommend this book not only to expecting mothers but to all women and their husbands or significant others.

Uzo Ihenko, Ph.D
President/CEO
Uzo 1 International, Ltd
Buffalo New York USA

FOREWORD: 2

Eleanore Chillis and I grew up in New Hope Church of God in Christ during the 1970's. The Elder Ureese Chillis, her uncle, was the pastor. I always considered her an outlier and one of the most detailed oriented people that I have ever known. She has the phenomenal ability to critically analyze topics that most people would overlook.

Eleanore and I lost contact after I went into the military in the 1980's. About 30 years later (2013), we met again, by accident in my doctor's office. I heard the name 'Chillis' and asked her if she was Elder Chillis's niece and did she grow up at New Hope Church of God in Christ on Masten Avenue in Buffalo. She replied, "*Yes that's me*!"

From 2013 to the present, we have been working together in the Buffalo community to reduce poverty and sickness in African American neighborhoods. In 2014, we designed and ran a successful pilot program that addressed African American women's health relating to obesity. This pilot program led to the creation of our not-for-profit organization, LifeSource Systems, Inc (LSS).

Eleanore's book is not only timely as she shares the experience of birthing her son Kelechi but will allow other Black women to know that they are not alone in the fight to eradicate implicit bias and injustices. "*NOW, THEREFORE, I, JOSEPH R. BIDEN JR., President of the United States of America, by virtue of the authority vested in me by the Constitution and the laws of the United States, do hereby proclaim April 11 through April 17, 2023, as Black Maternal Health Week. I call upon all Americans to raise awareness of the state of Black maternal health in the United States by understanding the consequences of institutional racism; recognizing the scope of this problem and the need for urgent solutions; amplifying the voices and experiences of Black women, families, and communities; and committing to building a world in which Black women do not have to fear for their safety, their well-being, their dignity, or their lives before, during, and after pregnancy.*"

The United States Government. (2023, April 10). A proclamation on Black Maternal Health Week, 2023. The White House. https://www.whitehouse.gov/briefing-room/presidential-actions/2023/04/10/a-proclamation-on-black-maternal-health-week-2023/

So, as you can see, great strides have been made to bring this pivotal subject to light and what better way to gain an in-depth perspective than reading it from the author herself; for which I am elated to have a part in this awesome feat.

MHPMM speaks volumes for Black American Women and their lack of trust in the maternal health pregnancy arena.

Pamela James, MS, MA
CEO, LifeSource Systems, Inc.

INTRODUCTION

I don't know how many times I've told this story, probably at least 1000 times, and I wouldn't be lying. If it was an estimate that number would be closer to an exact number, then an estimated one. Just as compelling, during visiting hours, I would visit my newborn in the NICU. Either, I would sing or hum "*twinkle, twinkle little star, to how I wonder what you are.*" Thus, serenading all the infants in the NICU as well. I was discharged from the hospital without ever holding my son because I must have first been able to sit in one of those old ass rocking chairs. Due to the very little use of my hip flexors I couldn't bend or sit that low.

Incidentally, as soon as I was released from the hospital, I started therapy right away and had to learn to walk properly again. Neither was I able to see my infant for the first three days after delivery. I was being treated in recovery for severe pre-eclampsia and wasn't able to transfer over onto the required gurney bed while being transferred back to my fifth-floor hospital room. The fifth floor was for high-risk sick mommy's with pregnancy complications. Had I been transferred over onto the gurney they would have been able to swing by the NICU and let me see my baby through the window. However, that didn't happen either.

In 1997 or 1998 was the last time I sat and tried to write my story for future reference. My head hurt so badly, I'm sure my blood pressure went way, way up too. I cried and cried and the tears poured from my eyes like a cartoon character spewing water from his face/eye sockets, (lol). I vowed that if I made it through those feelings/episodes that I would not think about it nor attempt to write about it again because it was much, much, much too difficult to continue. Of course overtime, I told the story to others, though not with the same anxiety or intensifying purpose as before. I kept my emotional attachment shut off and at bay.

I became a very stoic personality type regarding this situation and so I closed off and to the point that I didn't follow, nor was I aware that such an implicit bias and pattern of not listening to Black American Woman was happening to others as well. It was the noise of Singer, *Beyonce*, Tennis Star, *Serena Williams*; TV News Analysis, *Bakari Sellers* and wife *Ellen Rucker Seller*; *Judge Hatchett's son,* Charles Johnson and *daughter in law*, Kyira Johnson, including *Sha-Asia Washington* and Olympic Medalist *Allison* Felix— I'm like, what the hell! Plus, many, many others all suffering a traumatic maternal pregnancy, morbidity or mortality issue of some sort.

At that time my knowledge and state of mind was very confused due to being a first-time mom and never being sick enough to have ever been hospitalized, let alone having a major surgery. In fact, the more I was learning about what was happening and the fact that it was still going on today is what made me revisit maternal pregnancy, morbidity and mortality issues in Black American Women.

The first time I ever heard about a mother dying in childbirth was at a friend's annual cultural gathering. It wasn't until after attending a number of events I noticed that I hadn't ever seen or met the mom. Out of curiosity, I asked where the mom was and was told that she had died in childbirth. I thought about how sad it must be for the children. Although I have never known anyone to have passed away through childbirth, I knew of women who have lost an infant during or after delivery or to SIDS.

I never intended to write this book, but knowing how important it is to compile data records, share our stories and make informed decisions, it became necessary. Using midwifery's, midwives and doulas as the alternative to eliminating the assembly line model of care and redirect the course of birthing equity towards better birthing solutions.

In an effort to share firsthand experiences when it comes to pain and not being heard or listened to, I therefore hereby forge through copies of my actual medical records and reports and take you through a documented maternal morbidity and survival. From the prenatal visits; early hospital admissions; surgical procedure, post prep and recovering anxiety, it's all here. You'll find that the epidural or anesthesia never appropriately worked. Read for yourself the intra-operative care plan, anesthesia charts and additional IV sedation given and do a cross analysis for yourself; along with photos and links to other informative reading material; for the sake of making informed decisions and knowing your maternal future risk always get copies of any medical records, surgical operative reports procedures and findings and utilize any and all appropriate paternal and maternal available tool kits.

As I've read and heard about the stories of others, I knew and felt in my heart that something wasn't right with my entire maternal hospital experience. At that time not being informed that all of what happened to me was an intentional or unintentional implicitness or a common ongoing unconscious bias practice towards Black women in America.

I never knew about implicit bias in healthcare or hospital disparities leading to maternity pregnancy morbidity and mortality rates. I never knew anyone who ever died during or after childbirth. I do know of SIDS infant deaths. I do know that according to a 1996 ABC News Report and transcript about how anesthesiologist drug addiction habits could be due to the readily accessible hospital/patient medication. I have a copy of the transcript that was part of my reading arsenal that accompanied me during my hospitalization.

(See Links: Compilation of fully related stories).

CHAPTER 1
HOW WE MET: 1993

The story begins in 1993 where we were both living in a downtown apartment for a number of years and never crossing paths. I lived on the seventh floor in a penthouse, and he lived on a lower floor. One day, while I was just finishing up a signature petition drive for the next upcoming mayoral race in Buffalo, NY, I walked into this guy named Uzo. He was the last constituent for the night, and I invited him to sign the petition. Uzo, an event planner, suggested that I come to one of his upcoming events at the Langston Hughes Institute. We bartered, if I purchased a ticket, he would then sign my petition. It turned out to be a win-win compromise inviting three or four others to tag along also. The rest is history!

CHAPTER 2
PLANNED PREGNANCY: 1996

After a few years, while Uzo was starting his Ph.D at the University at Buffalo, at the age of 40, I was planning a family with our first child. Prior to starting a family, I had always known that due to Buffalo's hot humid weather, no way would I have ever wanted a summertime pregnancy. To me all expecting mothers looked so hot and miserable while wobbling around in the summer heat. I felt that the extra body weight and effort it took to move about caused more heat suffering, than not! Especially for women who were much further along in their pregnancy. On that note! I didn't want my child to be born on two specific birthdays and thought I would choose my child's birth date month as well.

Of the two specific dates, one was my lovely mother's birthdate of March 9th as well as my beautiful niece's birthday on May 2nd. For no other reasons than personality types with my mom's zodiac sign being a Pisces and mine, a Gemini, I felt that that would not be a good fit. Not that I am, nor was I ever, a strong proponent of astrology or such. I just felt I couldn't stomach that difference. However, I do think it was mostly my stubborn ways and steadfastness in my thinking and nothing more than that.

As for my beautiful niece, not wanting to be obedient to adults, I just wasn't willing to put up with her ways simply because I didn't have to! I felt that I wasn't willing to raise a child or take a chance that he/she would be dismissive as such. But little did I know!

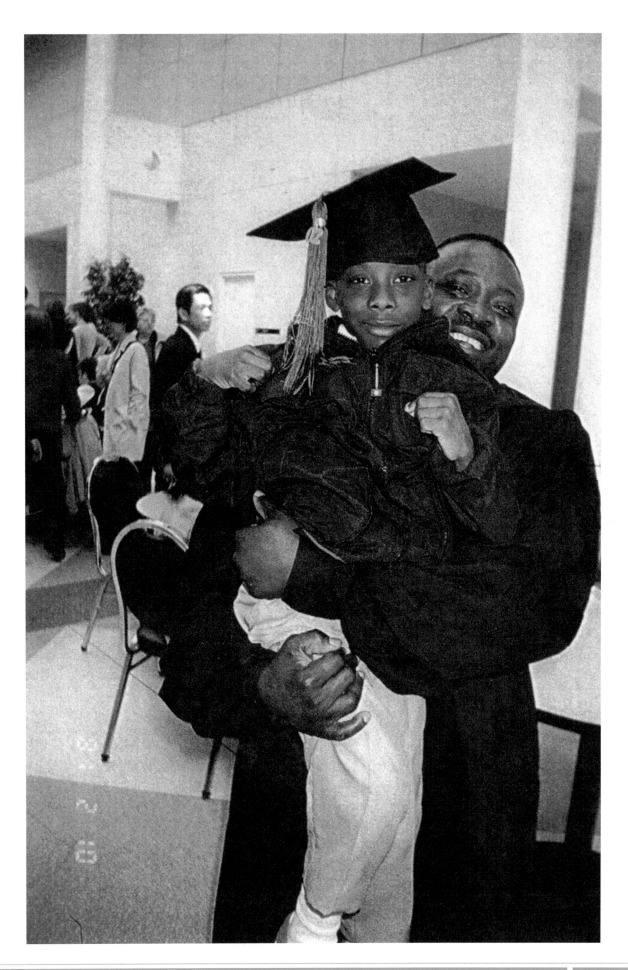

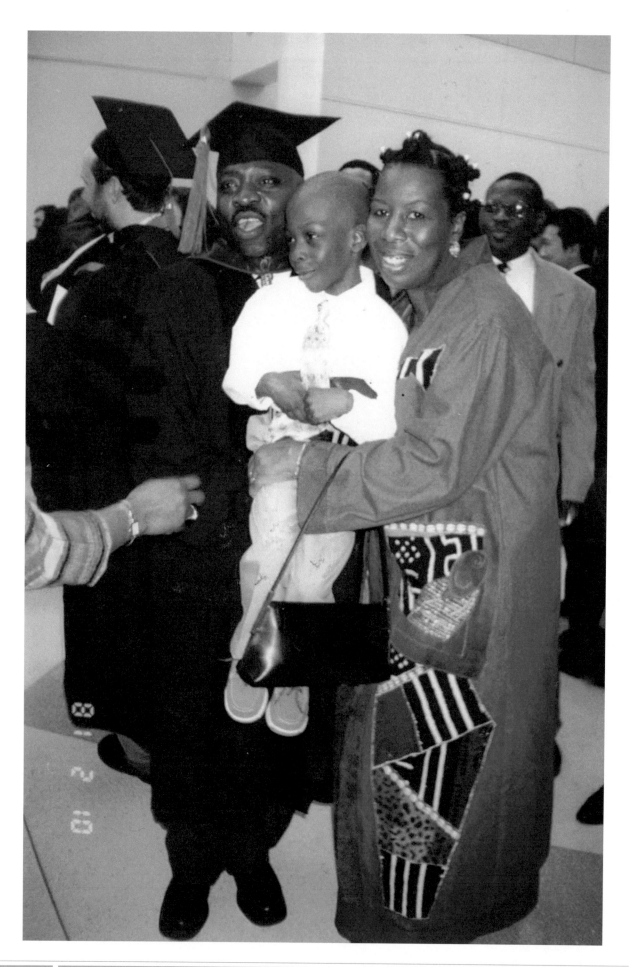

CHAPTER 3
CONFIRMED PREGNANCY AND DUE DATES: 7/24/1996 & 5/2/1997

My pregnancy was confirmed, and I'm told my approximate due date was May 2, 1997. You should have been there when we shared the excitement with my immediate family and were told that my due date was actually my niece's birth date of April 2nd. After the initial shock wore off and after repeatedly stating that her birthday was May 2nd, I gave into the fact that it was true and her birthday was actually April 2nd. All said, through the laughter and tears, I was laughing and crying every stitch of my makeup off. But wait, it gets better!

My baby was born two months earlier than my May 2nd due date at 3lbs 4oz. Y'all ready for this? He was born on March 8, 1997, 12 hours before my mom's MARCH 9, BIRTHDAY!!!!! YEY!!!! HAPPY BIRTHDAY MOM!!!!

I had asked if the surgery could wait another day so that my baby would be born on my mother's birthday, but I'm told after giving the last round of Magnesium Sulfate IV drugs the delivery had to take place within a certain window of opportunity for my survival and a viable birth delivery.

CHAPTER 4
PRENATAL VISITS:
1996 - 2/24/1997

It was very difficult for me to walk throughout my maternity and prenatal visits were the only time I would venture out. Uzo would prop me up from the driver side of the car and push me with both of his hands until I was leaning forward, then run around the car and pull both of my arms to help assist me out of the car. Basically, I was nearly immobilized, I would throw and drag my legs to walk while sliding my feet to maneuver.

Then, there was this awful pain on the left side of my groin that was bothersome throughout as well. Only to later find out that the cause was degenerating fibroids. Prior to pregnancy, I was never told that I had fibroids. I never knew because there was never any period pain, and like clockwork, my monthly was always regular. These issues were never addressed, and I thought this was just simply part of the Metamorphosis of being pregnant.

There is a lot to be said about the disparity and the lack of health care treatment for women, including a lack of investment in hospital labor and delivery floors and reproductive education for all ages. This therefore, affected the safety and the whole maternal experience and outcome, I'm sure!

Studies show that 40% of maternal deaths are preventable; oftentimes when Black women are complaining about symptoms and pain, they are not taking it seriously which turns out to be the cause of death.

The bias has no economic status, rich or poor; it affects African American women across the board. At one point in our lives, we all may have experienced the pain and suffering of not being listened to or heard. A clear and subjective pattern that continues today.

It's no secret that more Black women are dying even if they are more educated than their white counterparts based on zip codes, but more importantly, once at the hospital you are not taken care of at an appropriate level. In NYC disparities as a whole are 12 times more likely to happen to people of color in general.

Based on the disparities in childcare, if you go into the hospital to have a baby you could die. Dr. Neel Shah teaches reproductive biology at Harvard Medical School and works to build more equity and trust in the healthcare system stating that, "*What people are dying of is not the clinical condition listed on the death certificate, it is the failure of communication teamwork every time.*"

YouTube. (2019). *Closing the maternal mortality gap & improving outcomes for mothers*. YouTube. Retrieved June 1, 2023, from https://www.youtube.com/watch?v=kMZlfC0297s&t=10s.

As a Black woman, I too have witnessed such truths and have had a traumatic experience firsthand. A painful memory that still is emotionally etched in my mind today. Twenty-six years ago, there I was in a physically painful situation that was both dramatic and traumatic. As trauma unfolded before, during and after, I found myself lying in a supine position in the operating room (where as my fascial incision was being grasped with the Kocher clamps and sharply and bluntly dissected); in the effort to deliver my first and only child through an epidural anesthesia, cesarean, (also known as c-section), on March 8, 1997, at 12:15 p.m.

Patient's Name	Chart No	Date	Time
Chillis, Eleanore	2/49928	10/21/96	1145 AM

Address	Date of Birth	Phone #
10 7th St. Buffalo 14201	6/8/51	857-2557

☑ **PREGNANCY**

If any of the following signs occur, contact your physician, clinic, or return to the labor and delivery suite.

A. Regular contractions, (every 5-10 minutes) for one hour
B. A gush or trickle of water from the vagina.
C. Bright red blood from the vagina.
D. Sudden increase in vaginal discharge.
E. Pelvic or rectal pressure.
F. Fainting spells or loss of consciousness.
G. Severe or continuing nausea and vomiting.
H. Continuing or severe headache.
I. Swelling or puffiness of the face or hands, or marked swelling of the feet and ankles.
J. Blurring of vision or spots before the eyes.
K. Pain or burning on passing urine.
L. Chills or fever.
M. Rashes or sores in the genital area.
N. The passing of tissue from the vagina.
O. If you are 7 months pregnant and feel the baby moving less for a period of 8 hours or more.

☐ **BLADDER INFECTION**

A. Drink extra fluids (2 quarts a day), especially cranberry, orange or other citrus fruit juices.
B. Take antibiotics as prescribed.
C. Notify your physician or clinic if symptoms do not disappear in 24 hours or if fever persists more than 24 hours.

☐ **ABDOMINAL PAIN**

If any of the following signs occur, contact your physician, clinic, or return the the labor and delivery suite.

A. Severe or continuing nausea and vomiting.
B. Fever persists more than 24 hours.
C. Bright red blood form the vagina or rectum.
D. Severe or continuing diarrhea.

☐ **THREATENED MISCARRIAGE**

A. Restrict activity as instructed by your physician.
B. If any of the following signs occur, contact your physician, clinic, or return to the labor and delivery suite.

1. Abdominal cramping or contractions.
2. Bright red blood from the vagina.
3. Sudden increase in vaginal discharge.
4. The passing of any tissue from the vagina.
5. Return for second HCG in 48°.
6. Nothing in the vagina until next clinic app't.

GENERAL INSTRUCTIONS

Diet: ☑ Regular — *drink plenty of fluids. Eat a lot of vegetables fruits + bran.*
☐ Special:

Activity: ☐ No Limit:
☐ Limited to:

Medications ☑ Yes ☐ No

MEDICATIONS	TIME	SPECIAL INSTRUCTIONS
Colace	100mg tabs	Take one tablet twice a day (#20, Ø refills)

Special Instructions:

DISPOSITION

☑ Discharge — *Keep your next appointment.*
☐ Call your private physician to make an appointment in _____ days.
☐ Call your area clinic and make an appointment in _____ days.

I hereby understand and acknowledge receipt of the above instructions.

Eleanore Chillis
Patient

Witness

Physician signature

10/21/96.
Date

F-1871 (10/91)

If you have any questions or concerns, please contact you private physician, area clinic or the labor and delivery suite at 878-7035.

WHITE - PATIENT'S COPY   YELLOW - CHART COPY

CHAPTER 5
HOSPITAL ADMISSION: 2/27/1997

On Monday, February 24,1997, I was told there is a possibility that on the next well visit, I would be admitted due to the suspicion of having onset hypertension toxemia. A condition that could result in an early delivery, fatality or mortality outcome for both mom and baby. That week they sent me home with a Urine protein collection/test container and ordered bed rest until Thursday, February 27, 1997.

On the next visit, after a few days of bed rest and collecting urine samples, I went armed and ready to be admitted with packed luggage, reading material and all. Prior to my delivery due date of May 5, 1997, I was admitted to the Buffalo Women's and Children's Hospital for a total of 13 days from Thursday, February 27, 1997 through Wednesday, March 12, 1997.

Due to a loss of flexibility and inability to move properly, whether seated, standing or lying back, I apparently became progressively and noticeably slow. How ingenious, I thought, the Emergency Room attendants used the sheet roll method to mobilize me from one position to the other while in bed waiting to be admitted to the maternity unit. Yet, at the same time given my condition, it behooved me that the sonogram test ordered by the *Black Resident Doctor* had not been performed in a timely manner. This was crucial because every maternal pregnancy, precautionary measures and imminent findings could have been on the line for a safe and viable delivery.

In a wheelchair ride over to the testing room, the transport nurse was ever so gentle. She would watch every maneuver and the placement of her steps. I had first noticed her movement in the ER while riding through the door and over the threshold, floor drain, and again upon entering and exiting the elevators on each floor. Curiously, I asked, why? She said, "*to take all measures to avoid injury to the patient during transport.*" (See: Chapter 14, Wheelchair Mishap, after delivery).

As suspected, it turned out my amino acid/amniotic fluid level was low. At 31.5 weeks gestation, fetus size was at 28 weeks gestational growth along with my admission diagnosis status being:

- Hypertension high blood pressure
- Mild pre-eclampsia
- Loss use of hip flexors (a condition not fully addressed at this time)
- Condition for deconditioning legs

- Intrauterine IUGR with minimal interval growth
- Patient Medical History, Significance for degenerating fibroids
- Blurred vision
- Right leg edema

It was then I was admitted and immediately placed on permanent bed rest with bathroom privilege only.

DIRECTIONS FOR COLLECTION OF 24-HOUR URINE SPECIMENS
FOR CREATININE CLEARANCE TEST

1. Collect urine in a gallon bottle as supplied.

2. Be sure that the urine container has a label indicating your <u>name</u> and the <u>dates</u> the specimen is to be collected.

3. The bottle <u>must be refrigerated</u> during the collection period.

4. Start the urine collection at 8:00 a.m. by emptying your bladder and discarding this urine. Then collect <u>all urine voided</u> during the next 24 hour period. The last urine collected should be at 8:00 a.m. of the second day.

5. Bring the specimen to Women'c Clinic after the collection has been completed.

6. Blood sample for creatinine to be collected when patient brings in the urine sample. ▬▬▬▬▬▬▬

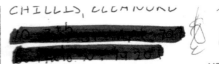

Obstetric Admitting Record

HOLLISTER®
maternal/newborn
RECORD SYSTEM

CHILLIS, ELEANORE
SEX: F
PA# 4704856

MR 2 14 99 28

ADM:02/27/97

Basic Admission Data

G	T	P	A	L		
1	0	0	0	0	L.M.P. 07·25·96	E.D.C. 04/29/97	AGE 40

Date 02/27/97   Time 12:00 PM
☐ Ambulatory
☐ Direct admit ☐ Transport ↓ ☐ Other ↓
☐ Wheelchair
☐ Cart/stretcher

Next of kin _____   Tel. no. _____

Reasons for admi.
☐ Onset of labor
☐ Induction of labor
☐ Spontaneous abortion
Cesarean section
☐ Primary ☐ Repeat

Observation/evaluation
☐ Fetal status
☐ Medical complication
☐ Obstetric complication
☐ Other _____

Detail reasons: R/O PIH

Patient Care Data

Contractions on admission ☒ None

Frequency ____ Duration ____ Quality ____

Began on __/__/__ at __:__ AM/PM

Membranes on admission ☒ Intact

☐ Ruptured: date __/__/__ at __:__ AM/PM

Fluid was: ☐ Clear ☐ Meconium ☐ Foul smelling

Vaginal bleeding ☒ None
☐ Normal show ☐ Bleeding (describe) _____

Patient has:
☐ Recent URI   ☐ Dentures/Caps
☐ Exposure to infection   ☐ Contact lenses
☐ Been vomiting   ☐ Glasses
☐ _____   ☐ _____

Plans for anesthesia ☐ None planned
☐ Specify type: _____
Last oral intake __/__/__ at __:__ AM/PM ☐ Fluids ☐ Solids

Allergies/sensitivities ☒ None
☐ Specify _____

Current medications ☐ None

Name/type of medication	Last taken	Check if brought in
PNV		☐
Tylenol		☐
		☐
		☐

Patient plans: (check which applies)
☐ Smoker ☐ Non-smoker
☐ Private ☐ Semi-private ☐ Rooming in
☐ Support person in labor and delivery ☐ Circumcision
☐ Breast ☐ Bottle feeding

Procedures ☐ Prep ☐ Enema (results) _____
☐ Other: ____ NC ____

Physician's name _____
Notified by _____
Date __/__/__ Time __:__ AM/PM

Significant Prenatal Data

Prenatal education

NO	YES	
☐	☐	Attended classes/received instruction
☐	☐	Received prenatal care beginning at the ____ week.
☐	☐	Records available on admission

→ Source of prenatal data: _____

Baby's physician _____

Lab findings ☐ None

Blood type & Rh	B+
Rubella titer	I
Serology	NR
HepBsAg	neg

Fetal assessment tests ☐ None

Date	Test	Result
/		
/		
/		
/		
/		

Latest risk assessment
☐ No risk noted at present
☐ At risk ☐ High risk

1. _____
2. _____
3. _____
4. _____
5. _____

Admission Physical Examination   Check and detail all positive findings

Ht.	Wt.	B.P. __/__

Temp	Pulse	Resp.

PELVIS ADEQUATE

System	WNL	Abn.	YES	NO
HEENT	☒	☐		
Breasts	☒	☐		
Heart and lungs	☒	☐		
Abdomen	☐	☒	pain over fibroids - palpable	
Extremities	☐	☒	LE edema	
Reflexes	☒	☐	⊕ DTR patellar	

Fetal evaluation
Fundal height _____
Estimated fetal weight _____
Estimated weeks gestation 31/2 weeks

Presentation ☒ Vertex
FHR 130-14   ☐ Face/brow
Station high ☐ Breech (type)
Effacement thick ☐ Transverse lie
Dilatation FT ☐ Compound

Position | | | |

Blood sent	__:__ AM/PM
Hgb	Hct
Urine Alb. ____ Glu. ____
Other tests

Nurse _____
Attending _____

Hollister.
HOLLISTER INCORPORATED 2000 HOLLISTER DR. LIBERTYVILLE, IL 60048
*TRADEMARK OF HOLLISTER INCORPORATED
OBSTETRIC ADMITTING RECORD   MATERNAL RECORD COPY

Health History Summary

Date: 2/27/97

PATIENT IDENTIFICATION

Patient's name: CHILLIS, ELEANORE

Home address: ████████████ STREET

City: BUFFALO   State: ███   Zip: ████

Age 40   Date of birth 06 08 56   Race or ethnicity B   Religion _____   Marital status _____   Years married _____   Education _____

Social Security number _____   Occupation _____   Work Tel. no. _____   Home Tel. no _____

Alternate contact _____   Relation to patient _____   Work Tel. no. _____   Home Tel. no. _____

Referring physician _____   Attending physician _____   OPTIONAL FOR INSURANCE, ETC.

Medical History

Check and detail positive findings including date and place of treatment. Precede findings by reference number.

	Patient	Family
1. Congenital anomalies	☐	☐
2. Genetic diseases	☒	☐
3. Multiple births	☐	☐
4. Diabetes mellitus	☐	☐
5. Malignancies	☐	☐
6. Hypertension	☐	☐
7. Heart disease	☐	☐
8. Rheumatic fever	☐	
9. Pulmonary disease	☐	☐
10. GI problems	☐	
11. Renal disease	☐	☐
12. Genitourinary tract problems	☐	
13. Abnormal uterine bleeding	☐	
14. Infertility	☐	
15. Venereal disease	☐	☐
16. Phlebitis, varicosities	☐	
17. Neurologic disorders	☐	☐
18. Metabol./endocrine disorders	☐	☐
19. Anemia/hemoglobinopathy	☐	☐
20. Blood disorders	☐	☐
21. Drug abuse	☐	
22. Smoking/alcohol use	☐	
23. Infectious diseases	☐	
24. Operations/accidents	☐	
25. Allergies/meds sensitivity	☐	
26. Blood transfusions	☐	
27. Other hospitalizations	☐	
28. _____	☐	☐
29. _____	☐	☐
30. No known disease/problems	☐	☐

Allergies: NKDA

Meds: PNV   Tylenol

████ H: #2 sickle cell trait

PSH: ∅

FH: ∅ breast CA

SH: ∅ × 3   Quit smoking 4 yrs ago

Gyn Hx: ∅ STD's

Preexisting Risk Guide

Indicates pregnancy/outcome at risk

31. ☒ Age < 15 or > 35	
32. ☐ < 8th grade education	
33. ☐ Cardiac disease (class I or II)	
34. ☐ Tuberculosis, active	
35. ☐ Chronic pulmonary disease	
36. ☐ Thrombophlebitis	
37. ☐ Endocrinopathy	
38. ☐ Epilepsy (on medication)	
39. ☐ Infertility (treated)	
40. ☐ 2 abortions (spontaneous/induced)	
41. ☐ ≥ 7 deliveries	
42. ☐ Previous preterm or SGA infants	
43. ☐ Infants ≥ 4,000 gms	
44. ☐ Isoimmunization (ABO, etc.)	
45. ☐ Hemorrhage during previous preg.	
46. ☐ Previous preeclampsia	
47. ☐ Surgically scarred uterus	
48. ☐ Preg. without familial support	
49. ☐ Second pregnancy in 12 months	
50. ☐ Smoking (≥ 1 pack per day)	
51. ☐ _____	
52. ☐ _____	
53. ☐ _____	

Indicates pregnancy/outcome at high risk

54. ☒ Age ≥ 40	
55. ☐ Diabetes mellitus	
56. ☐ Hypertension	
57. ☐ Cardiac disease (class III or IV)	
58. ☐ Chronic renal disease	
59. ☐ Congenital/chromosomal anomalie	
60. ☐ Hemoglobinopathies	
61. ☐ Isoimmunization (Rh)	
62. ☐ Alcohol or drug abuse	
63. ☐ Habitual abortions	
64. ☐ Incompetent cervix	
65. ☐ Prior fetal or neonatal death	
66. ☐ Prior neurologically damaged infar	
67. ☐ Significant social problems	
68. ☐ _____	
69. ☐ _____	
70. ☐ _____	

Historical Risk Status

71. ☐ No risk factors noted	
72. ☐ At risk	
73. ☐ At high risk	

Menstrual History	Onset age	Cycle q.	Length days	Amount days	LMP	07/25/96 quality

Pregnancy History	Grav 1	Term 0	Pret 0	Abor 0	Live 0	EDC 04/29/97

No.	Month/year	Sex	Weight at birth	Wks. gest.	Hrs. in labor	Type of delivery	Details of delivery: Include anesthesia and maternal or newborn complications. Use Risk Guide numbers where applicable.
1							
2							
3							
4							
5							
6							
7							
8							

Chillis.

CHILLIS, ELEANORE
SEX: F   , M.D.
PA# 4704856   DOB: 06/08/56
                              ADM:02/27/97
MR **2 14 99 28**

Admission Note

DATE	TIME	
2/27/97		40 y o BF G₁ P₀, LMP 7/25/96
		EDC 4/29/97 by R ult sono,
1250		EGA 31½ wks, presents c̄ 4 o
		H/A blurry vision, LE swelling.
		Pt c̄ h/o 3 degenerating fibroids
		c̄ excruciating pain all day.
		LABS B pos / R I / NR / (neg)
		P med Hx Sickle cell trait
		P Surg Hx ∅
		all NKDA
		Meds PNV, Tylenol
		FH ∅ breast CA
		Social ∅ X 3
		Quit smoking 4 yrs ago
		P Gyn Hx ∅ STDs
		⊕ pap
		PE BP = 136/82
		Rel see addendum
		FHR 130 - 140
		avg var
		⊕ accels
		↓ FHR, prob maternal ~~EC~~ HR
		Toco ∅ cntxn's.
		Sono Vtx AFI 10.1
		placenta posterior.
		BPP = 8/10 ⊕ FB ⊕ FM ⊕ FT ⊕ AF
		AUA 28 W 1 D
		EFW 1104 gms

24

PROGRESS NOTES

DATE	TIME	— Control —
2/27/97		Ⓐ ① IUP 31 4/7 wks
		② No preeclampsia
	AMA	③ Degenerating fibroids → pain
	↑ MSAFP	④ Desires PP Tubal
	Refused	███████ signed.
	amnio	⑤ ████████████████
		⑥ Baby measures small
	Ⓟ ① Admit
		② 24° urine
		③ T+C #3 prn pain
		④ CBC, sma 18
		⑤ Gc, chlamydia, GBS
		⑥ Preeclampsia precautions
		⑦ Monitor ███████████████████
		████████████████████████
2/27/97		Addendum
		Speculum exam attempted but unsuccessful.
	1335	Patient cannot tolerate speculum exam.
		Crx cultures not obtained.
		Crx = FT / thick / high digitally.
		███████████████

Form 32 Rev. 6/87

CHILLIS, ELEANOR   MR 2 14 99 28
SEX: F
PA# 4704856   DOB: 06/08/56
ROGERS, BRUCE, M.D.
ADM: 02/27/97

REQUESTED BY

DATE 2/27/97   V=9

REASON FOR CONSULTATION
PT for degenerative fibroids causing Ⓑ LE pain, also Ⓑ LE edema

☐ TEACHING CONSULT   SERVICE CONSULTED: PT

General Information: Pt is a 40 y/o B F admitted to CHOB on 2/27/97.

Medical History: Pt is pregnant EDC 4/29/97. EGA 31.5 wks. Pt was admitted to CHOB c̄ c/o HA, blurred vision, Ⓑ LE edema and has dx of mild pre-eclampsia. Pt is on bedrest c̄ BRP. PMH is significant for degenerative fibroids c̄ pain all day and sickle cell trait. [error PT 3/3/97]

General Observations: Pt c/o pain in Ⓑ groin area. Pt in bed c̄ external fetal monitor. Pt was attempting to change position from 1 side to the other and was moving very slowly. Pt alert and oriented, very talkative. Tolerated assessment well c̄ exception of hip flexion which causes pain.

Physical Assessment: ROM: Ⓑ hip ✓ limited 2° pain in Ⓑ groin area which does not refer down her legs. DF + PF WFLs. Ⓑ UEs WFLs. Strength: Ⓑ hip ✓ NA 2° pain. Observation reveals Ⓑ LE edema. Pt c/o Ⓡ wrist pain c̄ bed mobility + transfers. Pt Ⓘ in bed mobility but moves very slowly. Amb NA at this time 2° pt on bedrest.

Summary/Problems: Pt is 40 y/o F pregnant with mild pre-eclampsia and c/o pain in Ⓑ groin area limiting fxnl ability (bed mobility and amb as allowed). Pt is at risk for deconditioning, DVT 2° bedrest.

Plan: Introduced pt to TENS unit for pain management and

SIGNATURE CONSULTANT   X   DATE   TIME

F-0001 (2/88)

CONTINUATION SHEET

PAGE NO. 2

REQUESTED BY	DATE

REASON FOR CONSULTATION

TEACHING CONSULT ☐   SERVICE CONSULTED

left literature for pt to read. If pt agrees to plan, SPT will instruct pt in use of TENS and do daily checks to assess progress. Instructed pt in ROM exs for UE + LE. Informed pt of DVT signs + symptoms. Requested TEDS stockings from nurse for LE edema. Will provide wrist splints for pain in wrists c̄ transfers. Pt agrees c̄ pla

Goals: LTG: 1. Prevent deconditioning + DVT 2° bedrest.

2. Pt will be pain free.

STG: 1. ① in ROM exs. to perform daily

2. Pt will be ① in use of TENS unit if applicable.

3. Evaluate amb + need for Ⓐ.

⬛⬛⬛⬛ S.P.T.

SIGNATURE CONSULTANT	DATE	TIME
X ⬛⬛⬛ SPT / ⬛⬛⬛ PT	2/27/97	AM PM

F-0001 (2/88)

MEDICAL RECORD

CONSULTATION SHEET

The
Children's Hospital of Buffalo
219 Bryant Street, Buffalo, New York 14222

founded 1892

☐ CONTINUATION SHEET

PAGE NO.
/

CHILLIS, ELEANORE
SEX: F   RODGERS, BRUCE ?., M.D.
PA# 4704856   DOB: 06/08/56
                              ADM:02/27/97

MR 2 .4 99 28

REQUESTED BY	DATE
I/S	2/28/97

REASON FOR CONSULTATION

pt suspicious

☐ TEACHING CONSULT   SERVICE CONSULTED
SW/WHC

Pt. known to SW from pnc in
WHC.

Pt. has strong opinions re.
childbearing & medical care. Advised
her it is productive to be an
active member of her own
medical team & to ask Q. rather
than being critical.
Pt. feels care is excellent but
refuses to be an "experiment".
Advised her she would be given
full info. about all procedures
before anything is started.
Pt. has suspicious nature but can
be cooperative.
S.W. to follow & has my card.

SIGNATURE CONSULTANT	DATE	TIME
X ▓▓▓▓▓▓ CNTR	2/28/97	1245p

F-0001 (2/88)

MEDICAL RECORD

CHAPTER 6
BETAMETHASONE SHOT: (1ST DOSE) 2/28/1997

IN THE GLUTEUS MAXIMUS (BUTT): 1st Friday to help develop the baby's lungs, it was very painful. After that shot, every time someone came with a needle, it would cause me anxiety. From what I remember, I was given a 2-part shot divided into 2 separate weeks —Friday to Friday given shots into each buttocks, (a strong steroid to develop infants lungs to keep from collapsing due to early delivery).

— **What is betamethasone injection used for in pregnancy?**

   Antenatal betamethasone is primarily used to speed up lung development in preterm fetuses. It stimulates the synthesis and release of surfactant (2), which lubricates the lungs, allowing the air sacs to slide against one another without sticking when the infant breathes. injection:

— **A single course is recommended when the pregnant parent is at risk for preterm delivery between 24 and 34 weeks of pregnancy.**

— **A single course is recommended between 34 and 37 weeks for those at risk of preterm birth within 7 days, and who have not already received a course.**

— **A single repeat course of corticosteroids can be considered for those at risk of preterm delivery within 7 days, whose prior course was given more than 14 days prior.**

Steroid shots help speed up the development of your baby's lungs, & Miles, K. (n.d.-a). Betamethasone in pregnancy: How steroid shots can help your baby's lungs. BabyCenter. https://www.babycenter.com/pregnancy/your-body/should-i-take-steroids-during-preterm-labor_5437

For that whole 1st week stay in the hospital my body became very sensitive and painful to the touch and treatment of any kind, as one would imagine. The blood pressure cuff was like a permanent fixture attached to my legs during bed rest and while sleeping. It continuously checked for an escalation in hypertension pre-eclampsia and edema. It would pump up, squeeze and deflate around the clock. It was excruciatingly painful and would hurt due to all the edema swelling. It brought on such tremendous anxiety that I dread having a blood pressure check today. The random movement of being monitored would cause me to wake out of my sleep, because it felt like something was crawling under the covers. The baby monitor wasn't any better. It was from old stock and would fall off of my belly constantly. I couldn't have had a good night's sleep if I wanted to. It was an ongoing effort, and the nurse was in and out of my room, throughout the day, all night and every night as well.

14

Enter Here
IN PENCIL
Number of
Forms in Use

CHILLIS, ELEANORE
MR 2 14 99 28
_____, M.D.
SEX: F
PA# 4704856   DOB: 06/08/56
ADM:02/27/97

DIAGNOSES _____

ALLERGIC TO: _____   DIET _____
(Record in Red)

Scheduled Medications

OR. DATE / INITIALS	EXP DATE / TIME	MEDICATION-DOSAGE-FREQUENCY-RT. OF ADM.	HR.	2/27	2/28	2/29	2/30	3/1	3/2	3/3	3/4	3/5	3/6	3/7	3/8	3/9	3/10
		Betamethasone 12mg IM & repeat in 24 hrs	7p	●	●												
		PNV & P.O. q day (Pt may take own)	8AM	X	●		●	●	●	●	●	●	●				
		Colace 100mg po qd	10AM	X	X	X	X	X	X	●							
		Colace 100mg po Bid prn	8am							X	●	●	●				
			8m								●						
		Betamethasone 12mg IM 2nd dose Betamethasone 12mg IM	8am		X	X	X										
			8am														
		Toradol 30mg IVPB q6° x24° (then prn)	445 am	X	X	X	X						●				
			1045 am														
			445 pm	●											●		
			1045 pm		X												

3/6/97 — MgSO4 3gm hr maintenance 1:05pm IVPB

USE RED ASTERISK *TO INDICATE DOSES
NOT GIVEN - EXPLAIN IN NURSE'S NOTES

Single Orders + Pre-Operatives

OR. DATE / INITIALS	MEDICATION-DOSAGE-RT. OF ADM	TO BE GIVEN DATE	TIME	NURSE INITIAL	OR. DATE / INITIALS	MEDICATION-DOSAGE-RT. OF ADM	TO BE GIVEN DATE	TIME	NURSE INITIAL
	Seconal 100mg po x 1 now	2/28	1:45 am			Tylenol ii po	3/7	2p	
3/6/97	MgSO4 6gm load IVPB	3/6/97	10:50p - 11:50p			Tylenol ii po	3/7	8p	

AGE _____ RELIGION _____ DOCTOR _____ DATE/TIME ADMITTED _____

25

PARENTERAL FLUID RECORD

DATE 3/7/97   ROOM 309

SITE _____

PUMP _____ CONTROLLER _____ GRAVITY _____

TUBING CHANGED: TIME _____ INITIALS _____

CHILLIS, ELEANORE
SEX: F
PA# 4704856   DOB: 06/08/56
MR 2 14 99 28
_____ ., M.D.
ADM: 02/27/97

TIME AM or PM	ORDERED RATE (CC/HR.)	SOLUTION/ADDITIVE	READING	AMOUNT ABSORBED	CUMULATIVE TOTAL	SITE APPEARANCE	CHECKED BY
11p	67	D5RL	0	0	0	n	ec
12A	"	"	63	63	63		
1A	"	"	135	72	135		
2A	"	"	199	64	199		
3+	"	"	265	66	265		
4A	"	"	330	65	330		
5A	67cc	"	400	70	400		
1p+	"		465	65	465		
8Am	67cc/hr		605	140	605	n/s	
930Am			690	85	690	n/s	
10Am	↑1000 cc L/R		719	29	719	n/s	
1040Am	off pump bag	150	68	767	n/s	
12pm	blu pit added	500	350	1119	n/s	
1250pm	↑1000 cc L/R ccpit	0	500	1619	n/s	
130pm	↑1000 cc L/R	773	—	2619	n/s.	
2pm		837	64	2683	n/s	
4pm	67cc° pumped cleared	891 0	54	2737 0	N.S	
5p	↓500cc° (tubing..)	50	50	50	NS	
630p	"	"	115	65	115	NS	
730p	50cc°	"	170	55	170	NS	
800p	"	"	222	52	222	NS	
930p	"	"	268	146	268	NS	
1030p	50cc°	"	323	55	323	NS	
12a			381	58	381		
				24 HOUR TOTAL			

USE A NEW FACT SHEET EACH DAY AT 11 PM

IV SITE APPEARANCE		INITIALS	SIGNATURE	INITIALS	SIGNATURE
N – INFUSING WELL	E = EDEMATOUS				
F – FLUSHING EASILY	R – REDDENED				
S – SOFT	I = INFILTRATED				
W – WHITE	DC – DISCONTINUED				

F170 Rev 4/85

CHAPTER 7
AMNIOCENTESIS: 3/4/1997

(According to the professional, C. C. medical. (n.d.-a).

"Amniocentesis is a prenatal test that can diagnose genetic disorders (such as Down syndrome and spina bifida) and other health issues in a fetus. A provider uses a needle to remove a small amount of amniotic fluid from inside your uterus, and then a lab tests the sample for specific conditions".

The Amniocentesis was performed the 2nd week Friday; along with the 2nd dose of scheduled Betamethasone including Magnesium Sulfate administered, otherwise one would be at risk for having contractions and possibly an early delivery, therefore, I initially turned down the first Amniocentesis test. As far as the Gestation period this was acceptable because the fetus was developed through an intra-uterine growth — meaning small. With the baby's lungs not being fully developed, it would also require caffeine to help keep the lungs from collapsing. That night I was having pain in my lower back. The nurse should have put a call in to labor and delivery if there were any signs of contractions. She had not called, so it was not until the start of the morning shift any action was taken. I was then taken to the 3rd floor. Since there were no signs of contractions or leakage, I was taken back to the 5th floor.

AM-NI-O-CEN-TE-SIS /ˌamnēōsenˈtēsəs/ noun amniocentesis; plural noun – ses (-si:z) the sampling of amniotic fluid using a hollow needle inserted into the uterus, through the abdomen to screen for developmental abnormalities in a fetus. Cook EchoTip Disposable Amniocentesis Needles Manufacturer: Cook Inc Used for aspiration of fluid from the amniotic sac.

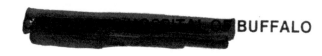 **BUFFALO**

DATE	TIME	
3/4/97		ROC
	01:45	S - Called to see pt re uterine contractions. Pt states this is new pain for her. She reports that she has had contractions starting in the afternoon, at 8 pm they became stronger, pt was medicated c̄ Tylenol but never monitored. Now pt is more uncomfortable. ∅ vaginal bleeding or leakage of fluid. ∅ HA, blurry vision, dizziness.
		O BP 141/82
		FHR 130s ave variability mild variable x_ ∅ accels toco q 2-6 min
		abd ⊕ palpable ctx mild - mod. ⊕ palpable fibroids cervix FT / thick / high
		A. IUP @ 31 6/7 wks gestation, mild preeclampsia Now c̄ preterm contractions ∅ cervical change Pt c̄ known degenerating fibroids
		IUGR vs. SGA S/P betamethasone 2/27 - 3/2
		P - Will transfer to L&D for closer observation Discussed c̄ Pt. _____
3/4/97		Progress note
	3:00p	S/ Comfortable still feels uncomf ctx but better
		O/ 35s FHR 130s any variable 145/78 uncomf mild variable decel 86 ctx not readily able
		A/ 31 6/7 wk IUP mild hypertens SGF vs IUGR mild preeclampsia

Form 32 Rev. 6/87

DATE	TIME	
		P/ _[illegible]_
		▓▓▓▓▓▓▓▓
3/4/97		Progress Note
	5:30 pm	S) Pt _[illegible]_
		O) _[illegible]_ 151/83
		[illegible]
		[illegible]
		Cx _[illegible]_
		P/ _[illegible]_
		[illegible]
		[illegible]
		[illegible]
		P/ _[illegible]_
		[illegible]
		▓▓▓▓▓▓▓▓

Form 32 Rev. 6/87

AMNIOCENTESIS TUBE/NEEDLES

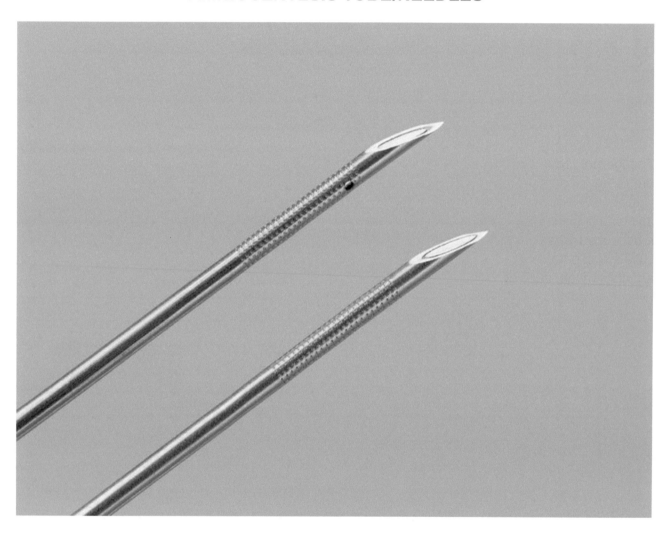

Products. Cook Medical. (2021a, May 13).
https://www.cookmedical.com/products/wh_dan_webds/

CHAPTER 8
THE NIGHT BEFORE THE EPIDURAL: 3/7/1997

Though not too disturbing to me, that night while I was in the Labor and Delivery unit with my own problematic concerns I overheard someone crying and hollering out for an extended period of time. Curiously, I asked the attending nurse whether someone was in labor and having her baby. I was later told that a nurse had experienced a miscarriage. Although her outcome was very sad, I didn't dwell on it because I was too sick myself, experiencing severe eclampsia and being treated with magnesium sulfate and betamethasone. However, I was more in awed, because the next day after the nurse had an miscarriage, she was back on the floor at work during my care. I don't know how she did it or was even allowed, but somehow, she was there!

CHAPTER 9

BETAMETHASONE SHOT (2ND DOSE): 3/7/1997

IN THE GLUTEUS MAXIMUS (BUTT): 2nd Friday **t**o help develop the baby's lungs, it was very painful. After that shot, every time someone came with a needle, it would cause me anxiety.

Benefits of steroid shots

ACS treatment speeds up your baby's lung development by prompting the cells in the lungs to produce a chemical called surfactant. Surfactant is normally produced by lung tissue in the mid- to-late third trimester. This surfactant production helps accelerate lung maturation and prevents neonatal respiratory distress syndrome (RDS) which affects a baby's breathing.

Steroid shots also reduce the chance your baby will have some other health problems, such as:

Neonatal mortality (death) in the first 48 hours
Bleeding in the brain, or intraventricular hemorrhage (IVH)
Systemic infection
Necrotizing enterocolitis (NEC), which affects a baby's intestines

Steroid shots help speed up the development of your baby's lungs, & Miles, K. (n.d.-a). Betamethasone in pregnancy: How steroid shots can help your baby's lungs. BabyCenter. https://www.babycenter.com/pregnancy/your-body/should-i-take-steroids-during-preterm-labor_5437

CHAPTER 10
MAGNESIUM SULFATE: 3/7/1997 - 3/9/1997

The use of magnesium sulfate to prevent or delay preterm birth can give medical professionals the time they need to prepare a preterm baby for the stress of the delivery process. During this time, physicians may administer prenatal steroids like betamethasone, which acts as a neuroprotector and helps the baby's lungs develop in preparation for life outside the womb. Being treated for severe eclampsia hypertension I was given 2 or 3 treatments; 7 - 12 hours apart, and then for another 24 hours after delivery.

The first dose was given through an IV tube the night before I was to go through an epidural anesthesia cesarean on the 8th of March. The Hep catheter in my right hand hurt all night, so I cried all night. Not only did the magnesium sulfate hurt, it actually had a burning sensation and caused me a sickly feeling. "*So still I cried.*" If memory serves me correctly, I believe the site of the needle went under the skin and was not properly in a vein or some of the magnesium sulfate dripped under the skin and had to be adjusted. My whole body felt like it was burning and my entire hand and lower arm was affected as it rendered my arm helpless. I kept my arm and hand resting on my chest for comfort.

I'm not sure, but all I remember is that something happened that night. The next morning, I made my way over to the bathroom. I used the call button for something, I don't quite remember, and the nurse came running because she thought I was locked in there. I was told that I shouldn't be walking around because I could have fallen and was then put on complete bed rest, bed pan *and all*.

I think I was given another dose that morning sometime before and or maybe during surgery. The treatment was so very uncomfortable, and I wished for it to stop! Little did I know, after the birth, I was given another 24-hour round of this stuff in order to mitigate the severe eclampsia hypertension. I was then sent off to recovery and put on continual watch for another day and a half, I believe. I was so afraid in the dark with the lights off and the curtains drawn. All these were part of the process of lowering my blood pressure. I cried for the remainder of March 8 and all day on March 9. I was so upset and wanted to know what happened to me in surgery.

continuing…

INTRA-OPERATIVE CARE PLAN

POTENTIAL FOR ANXIETY

GOAL: PATIENT AND/OR FAMILY DEMONSTRATES DECREASED ANXIETY

PLAN IMPLEMENTATION:
- ☑ GIVE CLEAR, CONCISE EXPLANATIONS
- ☑ COMMUNICATE PATIENT CONCERNS TO OTHER PROVIDERS, CONVEY CARE AND SUPPORT
- ☑ REMAIN WITH PATIENT DURING INDUCTION

GOALS MET ☑ YES ☐ NO COMMENTS_____

POTENTIAL FOR INJURY

GOAL: PATIENT WILL REMAIN FREE FROM INJURY

POSITIONING: ☑ Supine ☐ Prone ☐ Lateral R/L ☐ Lithotomy ☐ Other_____

TABLE TYPE: ☑ Standard OR ☐ Fracture ☐ Floroscopy ☐ Ohio Warmer ☐ Other_____

POSITIONING AND SAFETY AIDS:

☑ Safety Belt	☐ Kidney Rest(s)	☐ Eggcrate Mattress
☐ Blankets	☐ Padding Between Legs	☐ Hiproll
☐ Sandbag	☐ Thyroid Pillow	☐ Stirrups ☐ Hanging ☐ Davis
☐ Pillow or Blankets under knees	☐ Spine Frame	☑ Arm Secured: at 90° or less
☐ Axillary Roll(s)	☐ Headholder	Angle on Arm Board ☐ R ☑ L
☐ Shoulder Roll(s)	☐ Sheepskin	Arm Secured: Across Chest ☐ R ☐ L
☐ Chest Roll(s)	☐ Ulnar Nerve Pad	Arm Secured: At Side ☐ R ☐ L
☐ Leg Holder (Arthro.)	☐ Jelly Donut-Head	Wrist Restraint ☐ R ☐ L
☐ Pressure Padding ☐ Heels ☐ Elbows ☐ Wrist ☐ Other_____		

Electrocautery ☑ #_____

Grounding Pad Manufacturer _CTMed_ Lot No. _HOO-0183_ ☐ N/A

Grounding Pad Location _R thigh_

Temperature

Hypo/Hyperthermia	☐ Cooling	Location
Blanket use	☑ Warming	_____
Convective Air Blanket	☐ Yes ☐ No	

Temperature

Probe Location_____ ☐ N/A

Goal Met ☑ Yes ☐ No Comments:_____

POTENTIAL FOR INFECTION

GOAL: MINIMIZE RISK OF NOSOCOMIAL INFECTIONS

PLAN AND IMPLEMENTATION:

SKIN PREP: **SHAVE IN OR:**

☑ POVIDONE IODINE SCRUB & PAINT	☐ ALCOHOL	☐ NONE	☑ NO
☐ POVIDONE PAINT	☐ DURAPREP	☐ OTHER_____	☐ YES, BY:_____

GOAL MET ☐ Yes ☐ No COMMENTS:_____

TREATMENT AND MEDICATIONS

IRRIGATION: ☐ N/A   **MEDICATIONS:** *OTHER THAN BY ANESTHESIA*

		DRUG	DOSE	ROUTE	GIVEN BY	TIME
☐ NORMAL SALINE	☐ ANTIBIOTIC_____					
☐ WATER	☐ _____					
☐ GLYCINE	_____					
☐ LACTATED RINGERS	_____					
☐ N/A						

URINARY CATHETER: INSERTED BY ▮▮▮▮▮▮ URINE APPEARANCE _clear yellow_

☐ ROBINSON_____ ☑ FOLEY _16 Fr_ ☐ SUPRAPUBIC_____ OTHER_____ AMT. DISCARDED_____ CC

PACKING/DRAINS: ☐ NONE TYPE:_____ SIZE:_____ SITE:_____

COMMENTS:_____

TRANSFER SUMMARY

OUTCOMES MET:
- ☑ DEMONSTRATED ADAPTIVE COPING
- ☑ NO INJURY OBSERVED
- ☑ INFECTION CONTROL MEASURES MAINTAINED
- ☑ PRE-OP SKIN CONDITION MAINTAINED

DRESSINGS:
- ☑ STERI STRIPS ☐ TELFA ☐ XEROFORM ☐ ANTIBIOTIC OINTMENT
- ☑ 4x4 ☐ 2x2 ☐ ABD ☐ OTHER_____

DISCHARGE TO:
☑ PARR ☐ ICU ☐ ICN ☐ PATIENT FLOOR

POSITION:
☑ SUPINE ☐ LATERAL ☐ OTHER

COMMENTS:_____

▮▮▮▮▮   3/8/97

MR#:   002149928
Name: CHILLIS, ELEANORE
DOB: 06/08/56
Surgeon: ████████████████████
Assistant: ████████████ M.D.
            ████████████ M.D.
Procedure Date: 03/08/97

Dict: ████████████ M.D.
LJG/12627
6514

Dictated: 03/08/97
Transcribed: 03/10/97

cc: ████████████ M.D.

OPERATIVE REPORT

PREOPERATIVE DIAGNOSIS: Intrauterine pregnancy at 32-3/7 weeks, severe pre-eclampsia, IUGR with minimal interval growth, oligohydramnios, degenerating fibroids, undesired future fertility

POSTOPERATIVE DIAGNOSIS: Same as above

OPERATION: Primary low segment transverse cesarean section and bilateral tubal ligation modified Pomeroy

ANESTHESIA: Epidural anesthesia with additional IV sedation.

FINDINGS AT THE TIME OF SURGERY: Viable male infant weight of 1476 grams, Apgar scores of 6 at one minute and 8 at five minutes. The cord pH was 7.23, base excess minus on and hemoglobin 14.9. The tubes and ovaries appeared normal. The uterus was noted to have a large left cornual angle fibroid.

PROCEDURE: After assuring informed consent the patient was taken to the Operating Room and epidural anesthesia was initiated, she was placed in the dorsal supine position with left lateral tilt. The abdomen was prepped and draped in the usual sterile fashion. A Pfannenstiel incision was made in the skin with the scalpel and carried through to the level of the fascia. The fascial incision was extended bilaterally with the Mayo scissors. The fascial incision was then grasped with the Kocher clamps and elevated and both sharply and bluntly dissected both superiorly and inferiorly from the rectus muscles. The rectus muscles were separated in the midline. The peritoneum was tented up, entered bluntly. The peritoneal incision was then extended superiorly and inferiorly. Then at this time the patient was noted to have increasing pain and pressure. Additional sedation was given to her by anesthesia. The peritoneal incision was then further extended superiorly and inferiorly. The bladder blade was inserted. The vesicouterine peritoneum was identified, was grasped with the pick ups and entered sharply with the Metzenbaum scissors. The incision was extended laterally and the bladder flap was created. The bladder was retracted downward using the bladder blade. The lower uterine segment was incised in the transverse fashion with the scalpel. The incision was extended bilaterally with the bandage scissors. The bladder blade was removed. The infant's head and body were delivered atraumatically. The nose and mouth were suctioned and the cord was clamped and cut. The infant was handed off. Cord blood gases and cord bloods were sent. The placenta was removed. The uterus was left in the abdomen and was cleared of all clots and debris.

The uterine incision was repaired in the running locking fashion in a single

CONTINUED. . .

layer with 0 Monocryl. Small vessel at the right angle of the uterine incision was noted to be bleeding. Hemostasis was achieved with three figure-of-eight sutures using 0 Vicryl. Good hemostasis was noted at that time.

Attention was now turned to the tubal ligation. The left fallopian tube was identified.   The tube was followed out to the fimbriated end. The tube was grasped in an avascular section with the Babcock clamp. The tube was doubly ligated with 0 chromic suture and transected.   The specimen was sent to pathology.   Excellent hemostasis was noted. The tube was returned to the abdomen.   The same procedure was performed on the right fallopian tube. Good hemostasis was noted on this side as well. This segment of tube was also sent to pathology.

The uterine incision was again examined and noted to have good hemostasis. The gutters were cleared of all clots and debris. The fascia was reapproximated using 0 Vicryl in running fashion, the skin was closed with staples. The patient tolerated the procedure well. A sterile dressing was placed over the incision.

The needle and sponge counts were correct X2.

ESTIMATED BLOOD LOSS: approximately 800 CC.

URINE OUTPUT: approximately 300 CC.

IV FLUIDS ACCORDING TO ANESTHESIA: Approximately 500 CC.

DRAINS: Foley catheter to gravity.

COMPLICATIONS: None.

The patient was taken to the Recovery Room on post partum ward in stable condition. Magnesium was started for her pre-eclampsia.

M.D.

Labor and Delivery Summary

HOLLISTER
maternal/newborn
RECORD SYSTEM

SEX: F   _____ ED, M.D.
PA# 4704856   DOB: 06/08/56
ADM:02/27/97

Labor Summary

G	T	P	A	L	Type and Rh
1	0	0	0	0	B+

Presentation   Position

- ☒ Vertex
- ☐ Face or brow
- ☐ Breech
- ☐ Transverse lie   ☐ Compound
- ☐ Unknown

Intrapartum Events   ☐ None

- ☐ No prenatal care
- ☐ Preterm labor (≤ 37 wks.)
- ☐ Postterm (≥ 42 wks.)
- ☐ Febrile (≥ 100.4°)
- ☐ PROM (≥ 1 hr. before onset of labor)
- ☐ Meconium
- ☐ Foul smelling fluid
- ☒ Hydramnios *oligo*
- ☐ Abruption
- ☐ Placenta previa
- ☐ Bleeding-site undetermined
- ☒ Toxemia (mild) (severe)
- ☐ Seizure activity
- ☐ Precipitous labor (< 3 hrs.)
- ☐ Prolonged labor (≥ 20 hrs.)
- ☐ Prolonged latent phase
- ☐ Prolonged active phase
- ☐ Prolonged 2nd stage (> 2.5 hrs.)
- ☐ Secondary arrest of dilatation
- ☐ Cephalopelvic disproportion
- ☐ Cord prolapse
- ☐ Decreased FHT variability
- ☐ Extended fetal bradycardia
- ☐ Extended fetal tachycardia
- ☐ Multiple late decelerations
- ☐ Multiple variable decelerations
- ☐ Acidosis (pH < 7.2)
- ☐ Anesthetic complications
- ☐ _____ IUGR _____
- ☐ GBS

Induction ☒ None
- ☐ ARM ☐ Oxytoc. ☐ _____

Augmentation ☒ None
- ☐ ARM ☐ Oxytoc. ☐ _____

Monitor ☐ None
	FHT	UC
External	☒	☒
Internal	☐	☐

Medications   Total dosage
MgSO4 2g/hr
_____
_____
_____
Time of last narcotic _____ A / P

Delivery Data
Method of Delivery
Cephalic
- ☐ Spontaneous   Type
- ☐ Low forceps
- ☐ Mid forceps
- ☐ Rotation _____ to _____
- ☐ Vacuum extraction

Breech
- ☐ Spontaneous
- ☐ Partial extraction (assisted)
- ☐ Total extraction
- ☐ Forceps to A.C. head

Cesarean (details in operating notes)
- ☐ Low cervical: transverse
- ☐ Low cervical: vertical
- ☐ Classical
- ☐ Cesarean hysterectomy

Placenta
- ☐ Spontaneous
- ☐ Expressed
- ☒ Manual
- ☐ Adherent
- ☐ Ut. exploration

Blood loss
- ☐ < 500 ml.
- ☐ ≥ 500 ml.
- Specify amount, detail in Remarks
(_____ ml.)

Configuration
- ☒ Normal
- ☐ Abn.
- If weighed: _____ gms.

Cord
- ☐ Nuchal cord x _____
- ☐ True knot
- ☒ _____ Umbilical vessels
- Cord blood: ☐ to lab ☐ refrig ☐ discard
- For: ☐ Type ☐ Coombs ☐ VDRL & Rh ☐

Episiotomy ☒ None   Suture
- ☐ Median
- ☐ Mediolateral _____
- ☐ Other _____

Laceration ☒ None
- ☐ ① ② ③ ④ Degree perineal
- ☐ Vaginal
- ☐ Cervical
- ☐ Uterine rupture
- ☐ Other _____

Surgical Procedures ☐ None
- ☒ Tubal ligation ☐ Curettage
- ☐ Other _____

Delivery Data (cont.)
Delivery Anesthesia ☐ None
1 =Local   2 = Pudendal   3 = Paracervical
4 = Epidural   5 = Spinal   6 = General

4 Epidural
IV Sedation
Administered by _____

Delivery Room Meds. ☐ None

		A/P
Pit		
1240		A
Pit		
1240		A

Chronology   Date
		Time	
EDC	4/29/97		
ADMIT TO HOSPITAL	2/27/97		A/P
MEMBRANES RUPTURED	3/8		A/P
ONSET OF LABOR			A/P
COMPLETE CERVICAL DIL.			A/P
DELIVERY OF INFANT	3.18	1237	A/(P)
DELIVERY OF PLACENTA	3.18	12 52	A/(P)

Infant Data
Apgar Scores

	Heart rate	Respiration	Muscle tone	Reflex irritation	Skin color	Totals
1 min	2	1	1	1	1	6
5 min	2	2	1	2	1	8

spontaneous respiration

Resuscitation ☐ None
- ☒ Oxygen
- ☐ Bag and mask
- ☐ Intubation
- ☐ Ext. cardiac massage
- ☐ Other _____
- _____ mins. to sustained respiration

Infant Data (cont.)
Medications ☒ None
- ☐ Volume expander
- ☐ Sodium bicarbonate
- ☐ Drug antagonists
- ☐ Umbilical catheter
- ☐ Other _____

Medications checked below were administered in the delivery room. Otherwise reference the Newborn Flow Record.
- ☐ Erythromycin ½%
- ☐ AgNo₃ 1% or
- ☐ Aqueous Vitamin K IM
- Admin. by _____

Initial Newborn Exam
- ☒ No observed abnormalities
- ☐ Gross congenital anomalies
- ☐ Mec. staining   ☐ Trauma
- ☐ Petechiae   ☐ Other

Describe _____

Basic Data
ID bracelet no. 33263
Hospital record no. _____
- ☒ Male   ☐ Female
Birth order: 1 (of 1 2 3 4 5)
Weight 1476   3#4oz
Length _____

Output
- ☐ Urine
- ☐ Meconium
- ☐ Gastric _____ cc (ml.)

Transferred:
- ☐ To newborn nursery
- ☐ With mother
- ☒ To NICU (in delivery room)
- ☐ _____

Deceased:
- ☐ Antepartum
- ☐ Intrapartum
- ☐ Neonatal

Date _____ Time _____
mo / day / yr.   A/P

Remarks:
pH 7.33   hse sds
HCT _____   Breast/Bottle
Hgb 14   hep - neg
_____

Pediatrician/Resuscitator _____
Attending _____   per _____
Date completed 3/8/97
Assisting _____

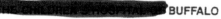 **BUFFALO**

SURGERY RECORD

CHILLIS, ELEANORE	MR **2 14 99 28**
SEX: F	RODGERS, BRUCE D. M.D.
PA# 4704856 DOB: 06/08/56	
	ADM:02/27/97

Date 3/8/97 Time Received 7³⁰A Priority: ☐ Elective ☒ Add On ☐ Emergency
Transportation _bed_ Or Case No._____ ☒ IP ☐ OP Operating Rm. No. (A)

PRE-OP ASSESSMENT

I.D. OF PATIENT: ☒ Verbal ☐ I.D. Band ☒ Chart

ALLERGIES: ☒ None Known List:_____

LABS: ☒ CBC ☒ HCT ☐ NA Other:_____
☐ Blood Type & Screen ☒ Blood Crossmatch Amount: — 2 units available
☒ CONSENTS ☐ HISTORY AND PHYSICAL
Skin Condition: _warm dry intact_
Personal Belongings/Prosthesis: _in room 304_

L.O.C.
☒ Alert/Oriented
☐ Sedated/Drowsy
☐ Agitated
☐ Unresponsive
PRE-OP MEDICATION
☐ Yes ☒ No

EQUIPMENT INSITU TO OR: ☒ None
RESPIRATORY ASSISTANCE IN ROUTE TO OR: ☒ No ☐ Yes _____
MONITORING DEVICES INSITU _none_
RN SIGNATURE ~~████████████~~ RN

SCHEDULED TIME	RECEIVED IN ROOM	ANESTHESIA BEGINS	SURGERY BEGINS	DRESSING APPLIED	ANESTHESIA ENDS	TRANSFERRED
to follow	11:35am	11:45am	12:15pm	1:30pm	—	1:40 pm
						to room 30

SURGICAL INFORMATION

PRE-OP DIAGNOSIS: _IUP at 32 3/7 weeks - severe pre-eclampsia IUGR, oligohydramnios undesired fertility_
SURGICAL PROCEDURE: _Primary low cervical pressure + bilateral tubal ligation._
POST-OP DIAGNOSIS: _same_

Surgeon's Signature ~~████████████~~ M.D.

Surgeon No. 1 ~~████~~ Surgeon No. 2 _____
Assistant No. 1 ~~████~~ Assistant No. 2 _____ Assistant No. 3 _____
Scrub Nurse ~~████~~ Scrub Nurse _____ Scrub Nurse _____
Circulating Nurse ~~████~~ Circulating Nurse _____ Circulating Nurse _____
Anesthesiologist ~~████~~ Anesthesia Resident _____ CRNA _____ SRNA _____
Perfusion/Other _____

TYPE OF ANESTHESIA: ☐ General ☐ Local ☐ Spinal ☐ Block ☐ I.V. ☒ Other _Epidural/sedation_

EKG Leads Location _anterior chest_	B/P Cuff Location _left arm_	Precordial Stethoscope ☒ Yes ☐ No
I.V. Line #1 Location _R hand_ Catheter _by R/O_ Solution _mg SO4_	I.V. Line #2 Location	Catheter Solution
Arterial Line Location Catheter	CVP Line Location	Catheter

PATHOLOGY ☒ Yes ☐ No Specific Instructions _____

Pathology Specimens:
1.) _placenta_ 5.) _____
2.) _R tube segment_ 6.) _____
3.) _L tube segment_ 7.) _____
4.) _____ 8.) _____

INFECTION CATEGORY: ☒ A ☐ B ☐ C IMPLANT ☐ Yes ☐ No CAST APPLIED Location _____

TOURNIQUET LOCATION _____ Applied By _____ Pressure _____ Time-Up _____ Time-Down _____

INTRAOPERATIVE LABS SENT: ☐ Yes ☒ No ☐ CBC ☐ Chem ☐ Bacti ☐ Blood Gas ☐ Other

COUNTS	SPONGE		SHARPS		INSTRU	
	☒ Correct		☒ Correct		☐ Correct	
	☐ Incorrect		☐ Incorrect		☒ Incorrect	
	☐ N/A		☐ N/A		☐ N/A	
IF INCORRECT: X-Ray Taken	☐ Yes	☐ No	ATTENDING NOTIFIED:	☐ Yes	☐ No	

COMMENTS: _____
_____
_____

Signature ~~████████████~~

F260 REV 6/9

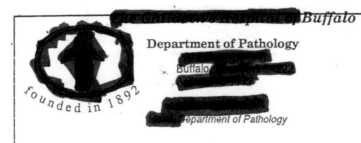

Patient: **CHILLIS, ELEANORE**
Case Number: S-97-01346
Medical Record Number: (0000)002149928
Account Number: 4704856
Age: 40 YRS Sex: F Date of Birth: 06/08/1956
Admitting Physician:
Referring Physician: M.D.
Location: VARIETY 5 0511

SURGICAL PATHOLOGY CONSULTATION

Clinical Information

32 week IUP pre-eclamptic IUGR, oligo.

Preoperative Diagnosis

33 week IUP

Operation

Prim. C/S BTL

Post Operative Diagnosis

Same

Specimen Description

A. Placenta
B. Left tube
C. Right tube

Gross Description

Labelled "placenta". Received fresh is a placenta with a 38.5 cm long x 1.1 cm attached umbilical cord. The placenta weighs 380 grams and measures 16 x 13 x 3.2 cm. The umbilical cord is inserted 2 cm from the closest margin and contains three vessels. The fetal surface of the placenta is dusky blue with yellowish tan areas along the margin. Grossly, there is no evidence of amnion nodosum on the fetal surface. The membranes are slightly opaque. The maternal surface of the placenta is ragged, red, soft, spongy, congested with grayish areas on its surface. On the fetal surface, there is a yellow slightly firm area measuring 1.1 x 0.5 x 1.6 cm. Cut section is unremarkable. Representative sections are submitted as follows:
A1 - distal end of umbilical cord and membrane
A2 - proximal end of umbilical cord and central region of the placenta
A3 - yellow slightly firm area on the maternal surface
A4 - random section of the placenta
B. Labelled "left fallopian tube". Received in formalin is a tubular tissue measuring 2.2 cm in length x 0.5 cm in diameter. After sectioning, the specimen is submitted in toto in one cassette.
C. Labelled "right fallopian tube". Received in formalin is a tubular tissue measuring 2.5 cm in length x 0.5 cm in diameter. After sectioning, the specimen is submitted in toto in one cassette.

3/11/97

Microscopic Description

6 H&E

Patient: **CHILLIS, ELEANORE**
Specimen Date: 03/08/97
Specimen Received: 03/10/97 1005
Copy to:

Printed on 03/17/1997 at 0556
Page: 1
Continued....

F2058

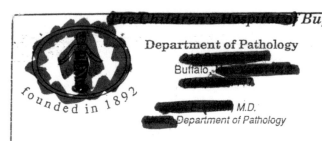

The Children's Hospital of Buffalo

Department of Pathology

Buffalo,

M.D.
Department of Pathology

Patient: **CHILLIS, ELEANORE**
Case Number: S-97-01346
Medical Record Number: (0000)002149928
Account Number: 4704856
Age: 40 YRS Sex: F Date of Birth: 06/08/1956
Admitting Physician: , M.D.
Referring Physician: , M.D.
Location: VARIETY 5 0511

SURGICAL PATHOLOGY CONSULTATION

<u>Diagnosis</u>

A. Preterm placenta with three infarcts
B. and C. Two Fallopian tube segments, unremarkable
Date diagnosed: 3/15/97

M29150, T88100, M54700, T86100

03/15/97

, M.D.
(Electronic Signature)

Patient: **CHILLIS, ELEANORE**
Specimen Date: 03/08/97
Specimen Received: 03/10/97 1005
Copy to: , M.D.

Printed on 03/17/1997 at 0556
Page: 2
END OF REPORT

S — Monitors Applied (IQ)H

Monitors applied. ~~████~~ started at 2gtts/hr. Elasticplast dsg ~~██~~. Foley patent & draining — urinary — ~~████~~
1:45pm — ~~██~~ ~~████~~ Morphine 7/2mg given ~~██~~ push by RN ~~████████~~. O₂ on ~~██~~ via ~~██~~. FOB and family ~~c~~.
1:52pm — ice chips given pt. Pt still ~~████~~ unable to relax. ~~██~~ ~~████~~
~~██~~pm — Pt still c/o discomfort. Demerol PCA 10mg dose given ~~████████~~
2:05pm — Dr ~~████~~ aware of ~~████~~ BP's ~~████~~
2:30pm — More comfortable — gd pain relief now. 3pm — Vss. ~~████~~ ~~████~~ well at 2gtts/hr. FOB at bedside. Sleeping ~~████~~

Denies Pain
Pt received asleep but arousable/groggy. denies pain. Denies visual disturbances. No epigastric pain. Lower extremities
— non pitting edema. ® wrist area ~~██~~

intact free of redness, swelling or pain. IV infusing per orders. ~~████~~
"discomfort"
awake & to incisional discomfort — ~~████~~ Repositioned to right
& appropriately. — NVPB Toradol but ~~████~~ per orders. ~~████~~ to ®
measured for TEDs hose ~~████~~ foleys patent for clear
yellow urine. Taking ice chips + small sips apple juice. IV fluids
~~████~~ ~~████~~ while pt taking po —

Sleeping intermittently. Reports good pain relief. Pt called RN to ~~████~~
check on baby. FOB ~~████~~ currently at the ICU. ~~████~~
Report given to ~~████████~~ LRN. ~~████~~
Report received from ~~████~~ @ L&D — Pt resting in bed. Offers no c/o @
present. FOB + friend ~~c~~. — ~~████~~

Pt arousable but groggy — ⊖ c/o HA, visual Dr, epigastric pain ~~████~~
dressing intact + dry. ~~████~~ bleeding noted. ~~████~~
comfort measures delivered — O₂ @ 2L 98% pulse ox sat. ⊖ c/o
@ present. FOB + friend ~~c~~. —
Pt resting in bed ⊖ c/o. FOB + friend ~~c~~ —
Pt sleeping (arousable) ⊖ c/o or s/s of preeclampsia —
O₂ @ 2L O₂ sat 97% VSS. IV site NS & infusing well. Pt
to bed.
Pt sleeping (arousable) offers ⊖ c/o @ present. VSS stable & cozy —
~~████~~
⊖ c/o visual Dr, epigastric pain. HA dry, I+E ~~████~~ O₂ @ 2L ~~████~~

3/7   12ᴬ Pt. in low Fowlers position, IV infusing Ⓡ hand retaped
      ∅ soreness.   MgSO4 3gms/hr via IMED pump, dynamap, EKG,
      pulse oximeter on.   O₂ cannula removed, SaO₂ remains stable. DE
12³⁰ᴬ Incentive spirometer given, pt instructed & used correctly
      Photo taken of infant in ICN — pt. very pleased c̄ first
      sight of son. ———————————————— DE   Knee high
      TEDS stockings on per order, no H/A, epigastric pain.
2³⁰ᴬ Clear liquids po.   Seizure precautions maintained.
3-4ᴬ Pt sleeping,   PCA Demerol available.
4⁴⁵ᴬ Ice, clears po. Deep breathing, leg + foot movement
      encouraged, → Ⓡ side lying position. Ketorolac 30mg IV
5-6³⁰ᴬ Resting comfortably ∅ complaint. Good output
      in foley. ————————————————————————— en
7ᴬ CBC drawn & sent, pt inquiring about baby
7³⁰ᴬ Pt talking on phone, pt comfortable.
9³⁰ᴬ Pt dozing. Encouraged use of inspiratory device.
10⁴⁵ᴬ Toradol 3[?]mg IV q6 given per order ⬚⬚
11¹⁵ᴬ Mg infusion completed and dc'd per Dr. ▓▓▓▓ ⬚⬚
12⁴⁵ₚ Am care completed. Linen s. Pt moving carefully and tentatively, ANXIOUS
      About experienced pain
      about experienced pain. Pt comfortable. — No c/o other than discomfort
      from abdomen ▮
1⁴⁵ₚ Report called to US. Pt transferred via cart

What did they do to me? Why did I feel everything? I asked everyone I encountered. I think the whole floor knew my story. What was even worse than that, was that I should have been resting quietly, but I was so anxious and too upset to rest. You see -- I was fighting, even when I couldn't. Before I was transferred back to my room on the 5th floor a nurse came to me and asked if I had remembered what happened in surgery. I told her that I had remembered the whole episode and that pain medication hadn't worked. I was never ever drowsy or woozy. I didn't get the chance to ask her why she asked; nor did she say. I guess I was too medicated and exhausted to ask, *but, would I have loved to know why*?

Sometime that night the nurse brought in a photo of my newborn. This made me happy! Because of my severe illness and him being in the NICU, I wasn't able to see him. I finally got to see him briefly without ever having held him, on Monday, March 10, 1997. As it turned out, it was 6 days before I held him for the first time. You must first be able to sit in the old ass rocker chair before you are allowed to hold your infant.

…continued

CHILLIS, ELEANORE
SEX: F
PA# 4704856   DOB: 06/08/56
MR 2 14 99 28
., M.D.
ADM:02/27/97

PREOPERATIVE ANESTHESIA NOTES

AGE _40_ WEIGHT _197_ HEIGHT _5'5_ TEMP _____

NPO? ☐ YES ☐ NO EXPLAIN _____

HISTORY AND PHYSICAL REVIEWED? ☐ YES ☐ NO   HCG REVIEWED ☐ YES   ☐ NO   ☑ NA

DIAGNOSIS AND PLANNED OPERATION _GT 32 wks . PIH._

PREVIOUS ANESTHESIA EXPERIENCE _Ø_   LFT - Alk. ph. 182

PREVIOUS ILLNESS _Ø uterine fibroids_   SGOT   21

MAINTENANCE MEDICATION _MgSO₄ , INV_   SGPT   15
                                                                    LDH   215

DRUG IDIOSYNCRASY / ALLERGY _NKDA_   Gluc 145

CARDIAC DISABILITY _Ø_   T.b.l 0.3

RESPIRATORY DISABILITY _Ø_   Prot. 6.1
                                                        (mild)   Alb 3.0
OTHER (PER FINAL REVIEW OF SYSTEMS) _Ø pedal & sacral edema_
                                    no RUQ or epig. pain   Unc. ac. 6.1
FAMILY HISTORY _Ø look in hosp. blurred vis on admis_   Chol 203

DRUG/ALCOHOL/SMOKING HISTORY _fruit 4y ago / 13y 1/2 PPD),   PT/PTT 9.6/27.3

LABORATORY _PLT 171   Creat. cl 70.9_

WBC _8_ HGB _12.2_ HCT _36.6_ URINALYSIS _protein +2_ OTHER _24° protein 552 mg_ OTHER _Ø_

HAVE ALL LAB RESULTS BEEN REVIEWED? YES NO   ARE THERE ANY LAB RESULTS WHICH PRECLUDE SURGERY? YES NO

PHYSICAL EXAMINATION

TEETH (missing/caps/crowns/loose/broken) _____

COUGH _Ø_ HEART _S₁ S₂_ LUNGS _CTA_ NECK MOTION _FROM_

BP _146/90_ HR _____ RHYTHM _____ ASA STATUS 1 2 ③ 4 5 E   BASIS _preclamps & sec_

RECOMMENDED MANAGEMENT _Epidural /ass GA_ ANESTHESIA DISCUSSED WITH PATIENT? ☑ YES ☐ NO

SIGNATURE _____ DATE _3/7/97_ TIME _16:00_

POSTOPERATIVE ANESTHESIA NOTES

DATE _____ TIME _____ BP _____ P _____

SWALLOWING REFLEX _____ CYANOSIS _____ GENERAL CONDITION OF PATIENT _____

SIGNS OR SYMPTOMS REFERABLE TO ANESTHESIOLOGY _None due to anesth_

IN-HOUSE PATIENT? ☐ YES ☐ NO   DISCHARGE? _____ ADMIT? _____ REASON? _____

SIGNATURE _____ DATE _3/16/97_ TIME _____

F 1107 (Effective 7/1/93)

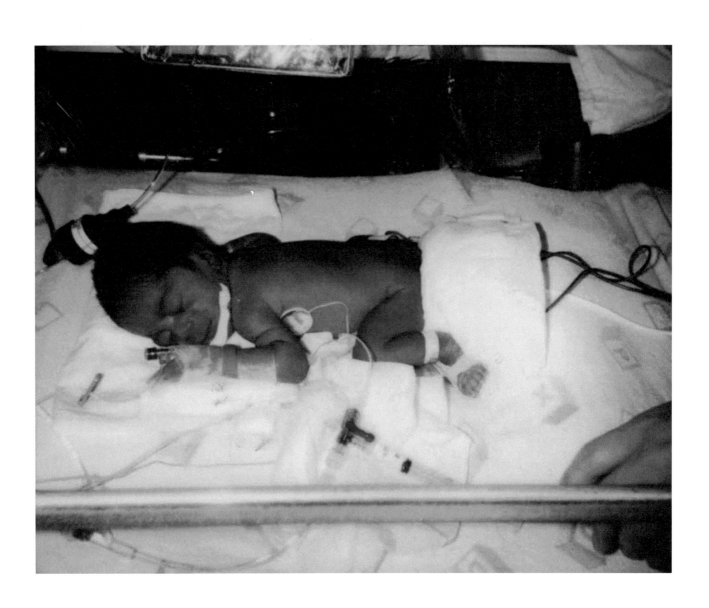

MAGNESIUM SULFATE: 3/7/1997 - 3/9/1997

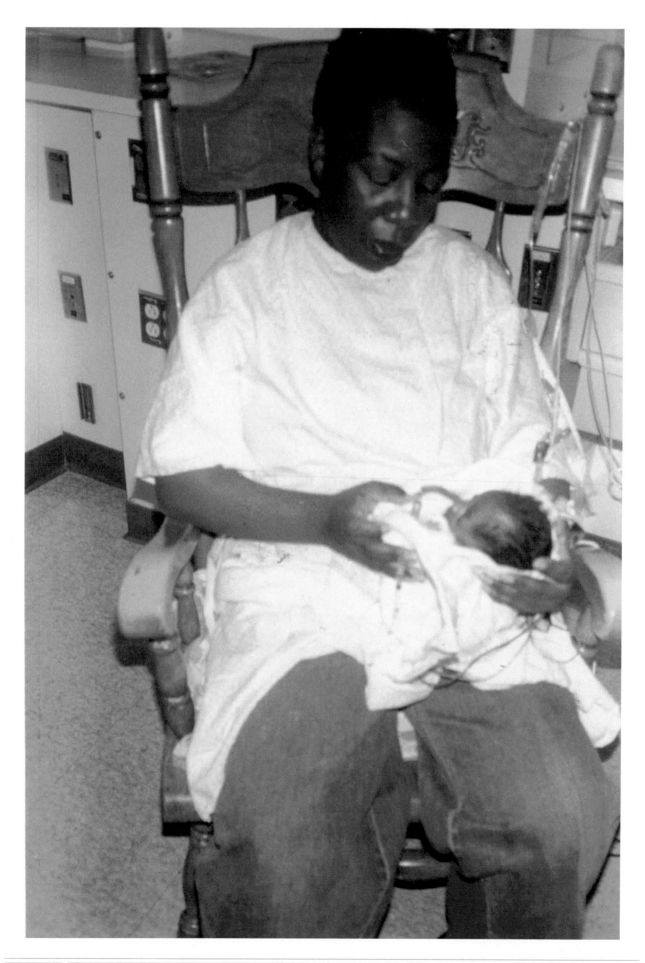

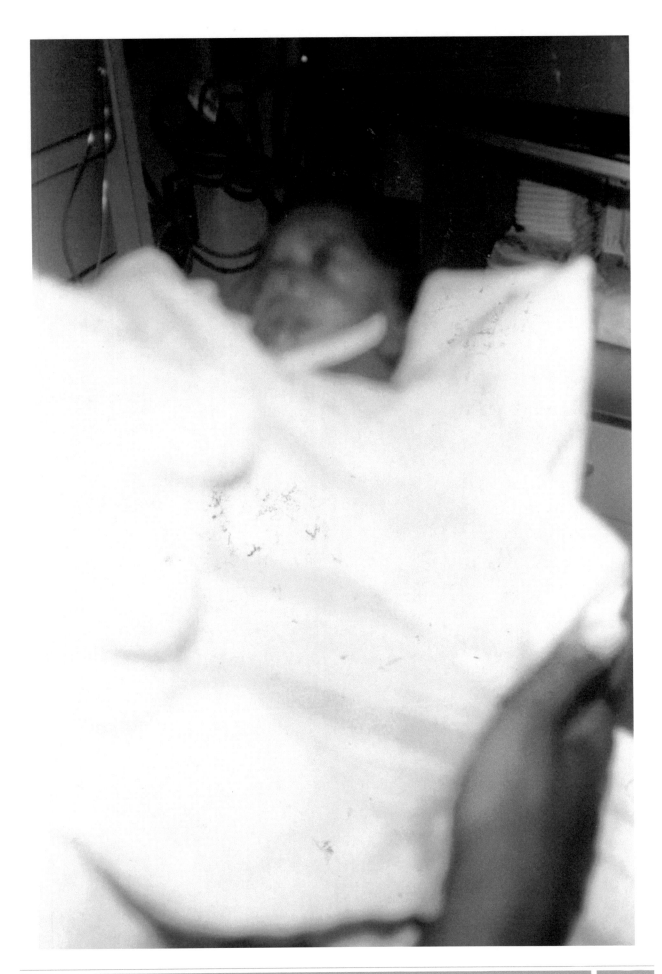

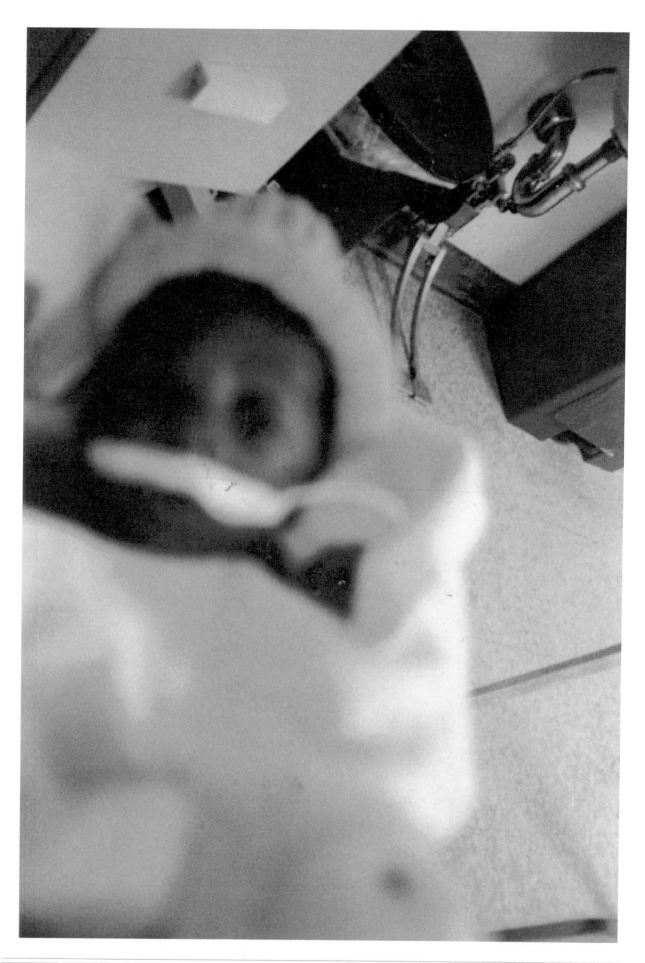

MAGNESIUM SULFATE: 3/7/1997 - 3/9/1997

ANESTHESIA RECORD

PRE-ANESTHETIC MEDICATION

CHILLIS, ELEANORE
SEX: F
PA# 4704856   DOB: 06/08/56
ADM: 02/27/97

DATE	STATUS	CONSENT
TEMP.	HEIGHT	WEIGHT

DRUG	DOSE		ROUTE	TIME
		MGM		
		MGM		
		MGM		

IDENTIFIED BY:
TAG ☑   OTHER:

ANESTHESIA PLAN FORMULATED AND DISCUSSED ☑
EQUIPMENT CHECKED ☑

MONITORING:

CARDIAC
- CON'TN EKG ☑
- CON'TN PRECORD.
- CON'TN ESOPH
- DIR. ART B.P.
- CVP
- DINAMAP ☑
- PULSE OXIM.
- CAPNO GRAPH
- O₂ MONITOR

OXYGEN L/MIN
N₂O L/MIN
% HALOTHANE
MG/THIOPENTAL 2.5%
RELAX

TEMP. PROBE:
- RECTAL
- ESOPH
- AXILLARY
- TAPE

SYMBOLS

EKG
FIO₂
SAT
ET CO₂
TEMP

B.P. ∨ ∧

PULSE ·

OPER. ⊖

ANESTH. X

RESP. BREATH SOUNDS
- INTUBATION
- POST POSITION
- FOLEY
- NG TUBE
- EYE OINT
- EYE TAPE

TOUR-NIQUET T

REMARKS #

Patient comfortable
Vital signs stable.

12:10 Incision made
12:37 delivery

SPONT. RESP. ○
ASST. RESP. ∅
CONT. RESP. ⊠

REMARKS # POSITION	
FLUID MANAGEMENT	
ESTIMATED BLOOD LOSS	

TOTAL URINE

AGENTS AND TECHNICS

TOTAL BLOOD
- ___ CC PLASMA
- ___ CC BLOOD CELLS
- ___ CC WHOLE BLOOD
- ___ CC ___

RECOVERY ROOM
- B.P. ___
- P ___
- RESP. ___

ENDOTRACHEAL: SIZE ___   ORAL ___   NASO ___   CUFF ___   PACK ___

DIRECT VISION ☐   "BLIND" ☐   AIRWAY ORAL ☐   AIRWAY NASAL ☐

OPERATION PERFROMED

NAME(S) OF SURGEON

TOTAL FLUIDS
- ___ CC D5 R/L
- ___ CC R/L
- ___ CC D-5
- ___ CC ___

- Fi0₂ ___
- O₂ SAT ___

SIGNATURE OF ANESTHETIST

PREOPERATIVE EVALUATION				BLOOD GAS				
HG.	HCT.	WBC	URINE	TIME				
				PO₂				
				PCO₂				
POST OPERATIVE EVALUATION				PH				
				BE				
				HGB				
				HCT				

FORM 114 (6/90)

[redacted]

ANESTHESIA RECORD

DATE	STATUS	CONSENT
TEMP.	**HEIGHT**	**WEIGHT**

IDENTIFIED BY:

TAG ☐ OTHER:

PRE-ANESTHETIC MEDICATION

DRUG	DOSE		ROUTE	TIME
		MGM		
		MGM		
		MGM		

ANESTHESIA PLAN FORMULATED AND DISCUSSED ☐

EQUIPMENT CHECKED ☐

Chillis Eleanore

MR 2 14 99 28

CHILLIS, ELEANORE [redacted] D., M.D.

SEX: F

PA# 4704856 DOB: 06/08/56

ADM:02/27/97

40-A

33

	12:30		13:00	13:30
OXYGEN L/MIN				
N2O L/MIN				
% HALOTHANE				
MG/THIOPENTAL 2.5%				
RELAX				
Versed	2			
Pitocin				

SYMBOLS: B.P. ˅ ˄ · PULSE • · OPER. ⊖ · ANESTH. X · TOURNIQUET T · SPONT. RESP. O · ASST. RESP. Ø · CONT. RESP. ⊠

Scale: 42, 40, 38, 36, 34, 32 · EKG, FIO2, SAT, ET CO2, TEMP · 180, 160, 140, 120, 100, 80, 60, 40, 20, 16, 12, 8, 4

REMARKS # POSITION

FLUID MANAGEMENT

ESTIMATED BLOOD LOSS

MONITORING:

CARDIAC
- CON'TN EKG ☐
- CON'TN PRECORD. ☐
- CON'TN ESOPH ☐
- DIR. ART B.P. ☐
- CVP ☐
- DINAMAP ☐
- PULSE OXIM. ☐
- CAPNO GRAPH ☐
- O2 MONITOR ☐

TEMP. PROBE:
- RECTAL ☐
- ESOPH ☐
- AXILLARY ☐
- TAPE ☐

RESP. BREATH SOUNDS
- INTUBATION ☐
- POST POSITION ☐

FOLEY ☐

NG TUBE ☐

EYE OINT ☐

EYE TAPE ☐

REMARKS #

ANESTHESIA RECORD

TOTAL URINE

AGENTS AND TECHNICS

800 mL blood loss
300 urine output

ENDOTRACHEAL: SIZE ___ ORAL ___ NASO ___ CUFF ___ PACK ___

DIRECT VISION ☐ "BLIND" ☐ AIRWAY ORAL ☐ AIRWAY NASAL ☐

OPERATION PERFROMED

C/S Tubal ligation

NAME(S) OF SURGEON

[redacted]

[redacted]

SIGNATURE OF ANESTHETIST [redacted]

TOTAL BLOOD
___ CC PLASMA
___ CC BLOOD CELLS
___ CC WHOLE BLOOD
___ CC ___

TOTAL FLUIDS
___ CC D5 R/L
___ CC R/L
___ CC D-5
___ CC ___

RECOVERY ROOM

B.P.	115/85
P	96
RESP.	16
FiO2	100
O2 SAT	100

PREOPERATIVE EVALUATION

HG.	HCT.	WBC	URINE

POST OPERATIVE EVALUATION

BLOOD GAS						
TIME						
PO2						
PCO2						
PH						
BE						
HGB						
HCT						

FORM 114 (6/90)

CHAPTER 11
ANESTHESIOLOGISTS: 3/8/1997

While being prepped I tried to tell the Anesthesiologists how I felt after the needle/shot was placed in my back. She didn't listen as I started to explain to her two or three different times. She wouldn't let me get any of my words out. She wasn't listening and didn't listen and was extremely antsy, swaying back and forth, moving about. She acted like she had ants in her pants, dancing and prancing in place. While I remained seated on the bed with legs dangling over the side, I thought this is *not* normal. Still not listening to me I asked myself what do I know? I've never had a child before so maybe this was normal. Although my mother and Uzo were both in attendance, neither one of them took note of this. Going into labor and delivery the Anesthesiologist asked repeatedly without listening to me, "*How do you feel and what do you feel*?" Even when I managed to blurt out how it felt (like cold water running through the veins in my left thigh), it still didn't matter to them!

Again, I managed to blurt it out and mentioned it to one of the attending nurses before the surgery procedure began. Still, nothing happened. In trying to distract myself, I could hear what sounds like dishes being washed, and I asked, "*who's washing dishes*?" At this point, I was placed flat on the operating table in a supine position with the table tilted laterally. The entire time they were hurting me. For months during my pregnancy, I was never ever able to lie flat, roll over or pull myself up from this position. It turned out my hip flexors (where the upper and lower half of my body connects) weren't working along with an increased buildup of anxiety. Then the Catheter was inserted. However, I don't think the situation with my hip flexors were ever taken into consideration with my arms stretched out at a 90 degree angle and tied down. Somewhere between here and there the doctor had already started the surgical procedure.

The surgeon started poking around and asking what I felt. Next, he started the first scalpel cut which was jagged because I moved. Then continued on with the procedure. Uzo was then brought in and I remember telling him to hold my hands that were both spread out far apart. I would cry out, hold my, and hold the other hand too. It's kind of funny now! He would run back and forth to each hand. I just needed something to hold on to. As a distraction, the Anesthesiologist asked what I was going to name the baby, I told her KELECHI. I felt she continued to ask, not knowing how to quite pronounce it, so I repeatedly cried out!!! KELECHI! KELECHI! KELECHI! KELECHI! KELECHI! KELECHI! KELECHI! KELECHI!

While feeling increased pain and pressure, the doctor stopped the procedure abruptly and clamped down, and stated that he could not get the baby because I was talking too much. When he would try to pull the baby out, I was bowing up along with him which I should not have been able to do. Therefore, he was going to call for the other doctors to assist him while putting me under additional sedation. Minutes later, what seemed like hours, I said to the surgeon, "*I thought you were calling for the other doctor.*" I then asked, "*WHAT'S TAKING HIM SO LONG?" and told him to STOP leaning on me so HARD; you're leaning on me HARD!!! GET OFF OF ME*!" I was then given the additional sedation. Once I was back in recovery and still in full blown pain, I was given a reluctant shot of Morphine because my body was already so loaded with many other drugs. Not sure what Toradol or Demerol is but it was also given to me after the Morphine for additional comfort.

I had to go to therapy for walking after delivery, but only after I inquired. They were sending me home in the same condition as I walked into the hospital with. This issue had never been completely addressed. Remember this was my first and only child so I wasn't aware of what care was expected other than delivering a baby. I felt pain all over my body before, during and after delivery while being dressed/cleaned up from surgery and then taking me back to recovery where I stayed for the next 2 or 3 days with a drawn curtain in a dark room. After the surgery, the Doctor literally had to help lift me from one bed to the other. The Doctor, though afraid because my body was loaded with drugs, gave me morphine because I was still in too much pain from the incisions. The Epidural simply did not work.

Pain Management Flow Sheet

Date 3-8-97 Room 307 Weight/kg _____

CHILLIS, ELEANORE
SEX: F _____, M.D.
PA# 4704856 DOB: 06/08/56
MR 2 14 99 28
ADM:02/27/97
38
25

☐ Epidural Drug _Demerol_

☐ IV Infusion/PCA Concentration mg/ 10 ml 1

PCA dose _____ ml Basal _____ ml/hr (continuous infusion) Tubing Changed: Time _____ Initials _____

Delay 6 Minutes

One Hour Limit 8 ml/hr

INITIALS	SIGNATURE/TITLE	INITIALS	SIGNATURE/TITLE

TIME AM/PM	PAIN RATING	RESPIR. RATING	SEDATION RATINGS	SIDE EFFECT	PCA INJECTED	PCA ATTEMPTS	BASAL	BOLUS	TOTAL MEDS. DELD.	NURSE'S INITIALS	COMMENTS
2pm	5	22	1	Ø	10	▨	—	—	10		Bolus dose hud. Morphine 7½ mg given
7³⁰a	5	19	1	Ø	76				60		
8³⁰	5	18	1	Ø	6	7			60		
10⁰⁰	5	18	1	Ø	7	8			70		
12A	4				1	1			80 mg		

USE A NEW FACT SHEET EACH DAY AT 11:00 PM

Pain Scale Used:

☐ Infants _____

☐ 3-12 y.o.: Smiley faces/oucher

☐ 13-adult: Ask pt. to rate or 0-10 scale

0 1 2 3 4 5 6 7 8 9 10
NO PAIN   WORST PAIN EVER

Sedation Scale   SS

0- No sedation
1- Mild (Occassional drowsy; easy to arouse)
2- Moderate (Frequent drowsy; easy to arouse)
3- Severe (Somnolent)
S- Normal sleep (easy to arouse)

Side Effects

N- Nausea
E- Emesis
P- Pruritus
U- Urinary Retention
R- Respiratory Depression

CHARTING KEY

F2011 (REV. 4/96)

43

Pain Management Flow Sheet

Date _____ 3-9 _____ Room _309_ Weight/kg _____

☐ Epidural Drug ___Demerol_____

☒ IV Infusion/PCA Concentration mg/ _____10_ ml _1_

PCA dose ____1___ ml Basal _____ ml/hr (continuous infusion) Tubing Changed: Time _____ Initials _____

Delay ___6___ Minutes

One Hour Limit ___8___ ml/hr

CHILLIS, ELEANORE
SEX: F   M.D.
PA# 4704856   DOB: 06/08/56
MR 2 14 99 28
ADM:02/27/97

INITIALS	SIGNATURE/TITLE	INITIALS	SIGNATURE/TITLE
██████	████████████████	██████	████████████

TIME AM/PM	PAIN RATING	RESPIR. RATING	SEDATION RATINGS	SIDE EFFECT	PCA INJECTED	PCA ATTEMPTS	BASAL	BOLUS	TOTAL MEDS. DELD.	NURSE'S INITIALS	COMMENTS
12A	4	20	2	.	0	6			0	█	
1A		18	1		1	1	–	–	10 mg	█	
2A		18	1		1	1	–		20	█	
3A	5	18	2		1	1			30 mg	█	
5A	4		1		2	2			50 mg	█	
7A	3-4	15	0		1	1			60 mg	█	
12N	4	24	0		4	5			100 mg	█	
3:35	2								120 mg		reset to zero
	2	22	0	0	0	0			0		
5:00	2	22	0	0	3	5			3		
6:00	2	22	0	0	3	5			3		
	2	22	0	0	3	5			3		
	2	22	0	0	3	5			3		
	2	22	0	0	6	8			4		
10P	2	22	0	0	(1)	(1)			(0)		reset

USE A NEW FACT SHEET EACH DAY AT 11:00 PM

Pain Scale Used:

☐ Infants _____

☐ 3-12 y.o.: Smiley faces/oucher

☐ 13-adult: Ask pt. to rate or 0-10 scale

0 1 2 3 4 5 6 7 8 9 10
NO PAIN   WORST PAIN EVER

Sedation Scale SS

0- No sedation
1- Mild (Occassional drowsy; easy to arouse)
2- Moderate (Frequent drowsy; easy to arouse)
3- Severe (Somnolent)
S- Normal sleep (easy to arouse)

Side Effects SE

N- Nausea
E- Emesis
P- Pruritus
U- Urinary Retention
R- Respiratory Depression

CHARTING KE█

F2011 (REV 4/96)

CHAPTER 12
ANESTHESIA: 3/8/1997

I was to be awake during the C-section delivery by Epidural Anesthesia. I don't know what I was thinking because I'm not *that kind of a brave person* but decided to go through with it anyway. I should have listened to my first mind as usual because it turned out that the epidural anesthesia did not do its intended job. *Duh!* According to the medical procedural report, I felt increased pain and pressure up to the point of being dissected both superiorly and inferiorly from the rectus muscles and extended to a peritoneal incision. At this time, additional sedation was administered in order to complete the delivery. (See: Inserted Operative Report Procedure that follows).

After the delivery, while being dressed, I continued to be in pain from the surgery (*crying out you're hurting me*). They could not lift me off the gurney onto the recovery bed. The nurses enlisted the help of the surgeon to come help out too. They counted 1,2,3 and hoisted me over onto the bed. All I could do was shout repeatedly, "*you're, hurting me, you're hurting me, I feel like I am going to fall, why won't my eyes open.*" At that time, when all was said and done while being transferred back to recovery, my youngest sister (Karin) the mother of three, said "*I never saw anyone coming out of labor and delivery hollering, it's only when going into.*" I said to her, Karin, they "*jacked me up,*" it feels like they cut me all over, (my feelings at that time). At this point, while back in recovery, I felt and knew that something wasn't right. I could still feel everything. I cried out and asked, '*why were my eyes closed and would not open, and why weren't the drugs working*?'

Again and again! I shouldn't be feeling this, the drugs should be working by now and I feel like I'm going to fall. I was just as alert and aware then as I am currently. I was never woozy or drowsy, I just couldn't open my eyes and felt like I was going to fall. I could hear my brother (Willie) asking from the hallway, '*what room I was in*'? Being quite alert I yelled the room number out to him. At some point while patiently and painfully waiting, I demanded they do something and had better do something right, NOW!!!!!! I shouted, "*I know the drugs should be working by NOW!!!!! I'm not even drowsy*!" Why?!

The nurse was running around frantically trying to get things set up, but I didn't care. Screaming, "*Y'all had better do something*!" I'm told she went running out of the room calling for assistance. The doctors and Anesthesiologist came and reluctantly gave me a shot of morphine. '*Can you believe they had to load me with more drugs*?' It was then my eyes opened. All together there were six other family members in the recovery room with me. I wanted to know why I couldn't see. (I think it is because I was in such pain, my eyes were shut tight). I was clamping down so hard, with a tight, fist, while holding on to the bed rails, to keep from falling. All the while visitors sat and watched. I was so mad and angry that such a thing could happen to ANYONE. Talk about an "*angry black woman*!" They just didn't know, oh how I wanted to do exactly, what I am doing now. Telling and showing the world for all to see.

CHAPTER 13
JOURNEY THROUGH THE TUNNEL: 3/8/1997

During surgery, I felt, I went to Africa and back (and still today, I stand by that journey as being real).

While going through the tunnel, everything was very, very pretty. It got brighter and sunnier still, the grass and the trees were green, and all the plants had bloomed. I said on my journey: Wow! Everything's so green and pretty here, and they said that Africa is so ugly, but it's not, it's pretty here. I can't believe how pretty! Then everything was moving really, really fast, I saw lights flashing, I saw dark shadows floating and moving all around.

I saw a wall full of concert vaults. There were people trying to send me back, I heard people calling me to come back/wake up, but on my journey, I wanted to see where the others were going as I intentionally and consciously looked back. I watched closely because I wanted to see where they were going and I wanted to remember when I had awakened. Before, turning back towards the voices telling me to wake-up. (Everything was moving and flashing really, really fast, lights were flashing and what sounded like doors were slamming).

While these dark shadows floated and moved quickly back into a specific vault as I looked on, one caught my attention, taking interest in me and got between us. As I was being called to come on and wake up, I first paused and said, ok, wait, I want to see. I consciously waited to see what was going on with the last moving shadow looking back at me, looking back at it. I believe what I then heard was the last vault close. It was so scary, but I wanted to remember this and tell others. I wanted to see if it was really true with what others had experienced.

When I came too, I said (confidently) "*Y'all, I went to Africa and back*!" The surgeon asked, "*What did I see*?" I repeated the above mentioned to the team — they laughed.

I told so many people first in the hospital, then at home. That I went to Africa and back. They probably thought I was crazy. I'm sure they really thought so when I reiterated it with poise, confidence and authority.

Once I was finally settled back in recovery and being treated with the last 24 hour dose of Magnesium Sulfate. I was still experiencing some flashing lights and large dark spots/blotches this time, bigger than the shadows. Being left in a dark and quiet room with no lights on, in total darkness as part of the treatment and healing process. Oh! How, I remained afraid during that time, because to me that journey was so real.

Although I've told the story about going to Africa and back, I've never given anyone the specifics regarding the shadows and the vaults.

CHAPTER 14
WHEELCHAIR MISHAP: 3/10/1997

Sometime, the night of Kelechi's birth, the night nurse brought in a photo of my newborn who I was unable to see because of my severe illness and him being in the NICU. I was so happy! I finally got to see him briefly without holding him, on Monday, March 10, 1997. I had 3 rooms in the hospital: 5th floor, (7 days), 3rd floor, Labor and Delivery, (3 days), and 3rd floor, Recovery, (3 days). Not sure of the exact order.

Meanwhile, while back in my original room, on the 5th floor, I noticed the other patient rooms were all empty. I took the liberty and borrowed the pillows from all the beds because I couldn't lie flat after the surgery. I needed to be propped up and supported. At that time, I was unaware that I had a hip problem. My hip flexor did not work. I also did not know what or how it connected to my inability to walk, sit or lie down flat. All I knew is that it was very difficult to stand up from a seated position or sit down from a standing position. I also needed assistance getting in and out of the car because I couldn't relax my rigid body.

In the meantime, while back on my 5th floor of the hospital, it was early evening when Uzo got off work. Although I was still very weak, and wasn't physically or mentally ready to venture out, he put me in the wheelchair and whisked me off to see the baby.

First, on the way across the door threshold, Uzo hit the BUMP and, oh LORD, I screamed a gut curling cry, so LOUD the whole floor staff came RUNNING. The doctors, nurses, including medics from other nearby floors in ear shot, as well. Although I had tears in my eyes, (while trying to keep everyone calm), I was laughing and crying out that I was okay. Mind you, I was still sitting in the wheelchair over the threshold in the doorway.

The doctor assured me that it was a common fear, the mom would think that her surgical stitches would burst! HOLY shit! The momentary pain was felt across the entire length of my incision, like a zipper pulling, from one end to the other. Both internal and externally of the wound. Though it was only momentary, it was very unsettling.

Secondly, I remember everything being so overwhelmed during my ride to the NICU. Running into and meeting the medical team, surgical doctor and other hospital staff along the way. Everyone congratulating me and wondering what had happened because they hadn't seen or heard from me after delivery. Some would say there you are, and others… *here she is*! Thirdly, moving on into the NICU meeting and greeting the caregivers of the preterm babies, who were too elated to have finally met me. While being wheeled around over to him in the incubator how shocked I was when they pointed him out to me. I asked, is that my baby? And the nurse replied, "*Yes, that's your baby.*" I then said, "*But I wanted a BLACK BABY!*" After looking at both Uzo and myself, the nurse said, "*Don't worry he is going to turn darker.*" I was like, "*Oh, okay, because there's no way I could do this again!*" That is, have another baby. (Truth be told… I thought, out loud, that's why I got an African, to assure that, I got it right the first time).

You see, even through the thick of it all, I still had GOD who gave me sanity and a sense of humor. That was my strength to get me through this ordeal. As I remained hospitalized I would even humor, sarcastically, at how I was jacked up during surgery.

During the conversation and ride over to my baby's crib side. My son responded to my voice upon entering the room by turning his head to the left side. I took note and alerted all others to do the same. As I continued on with the conversation and rode up on my baby to his right side, he then turned his head to the right following my voice. Everyone was so amazed that he had apparently remembered my voice.

However, years ago, I had this same experience with my infant nephew Kevin. When my sister Janet and I entered my mom's house yapping and laughing; he turned and looked at me with a full-on expression to show that he knew that voice. What an extraordinary experience that was! I'm sure it was brought on by the fact that Kevin's mom Karin both lived in the same household during her pregnancy with him.

Back to the subject at hand, due to the overwhelming anxiety of the day's events the visit with my son was brief.

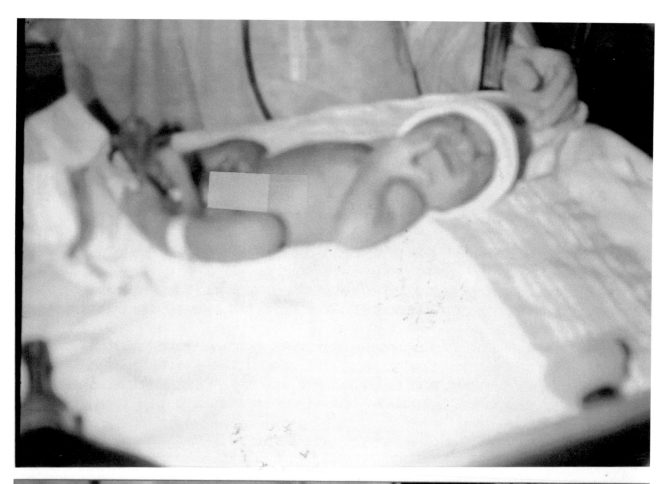

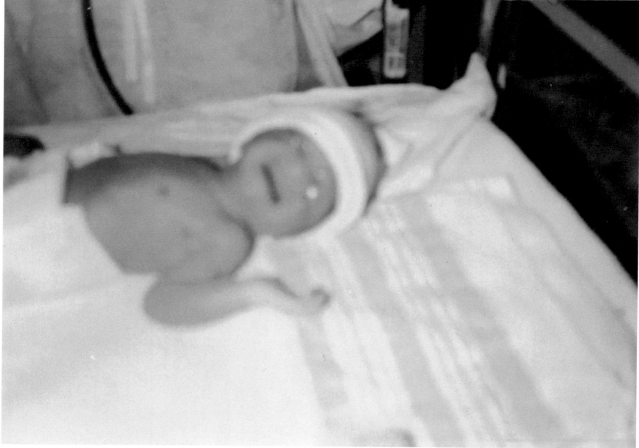

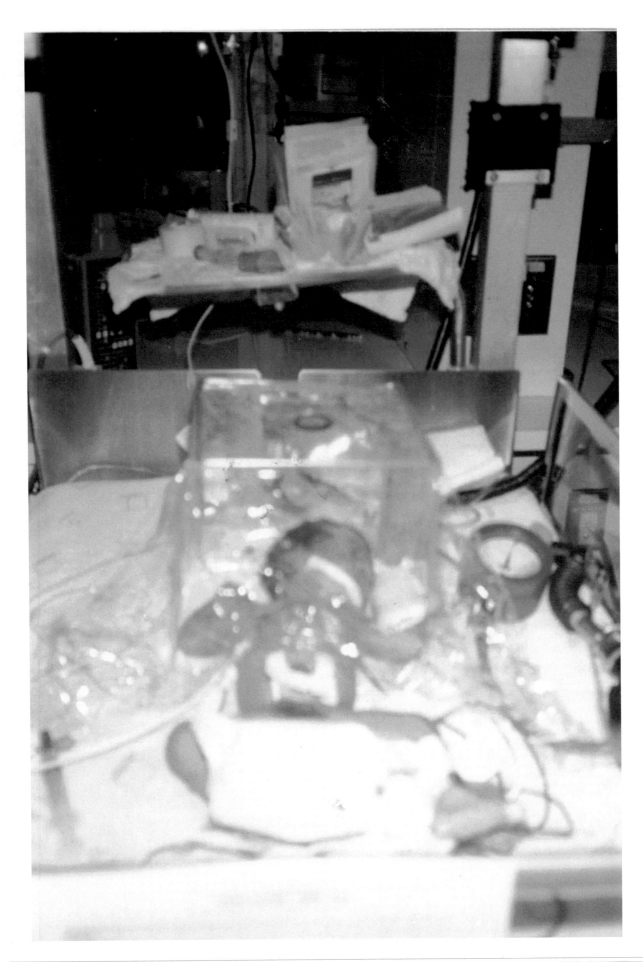

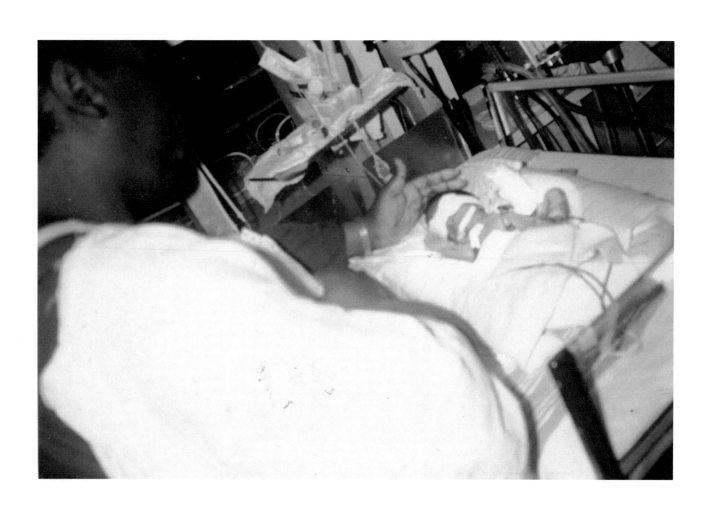

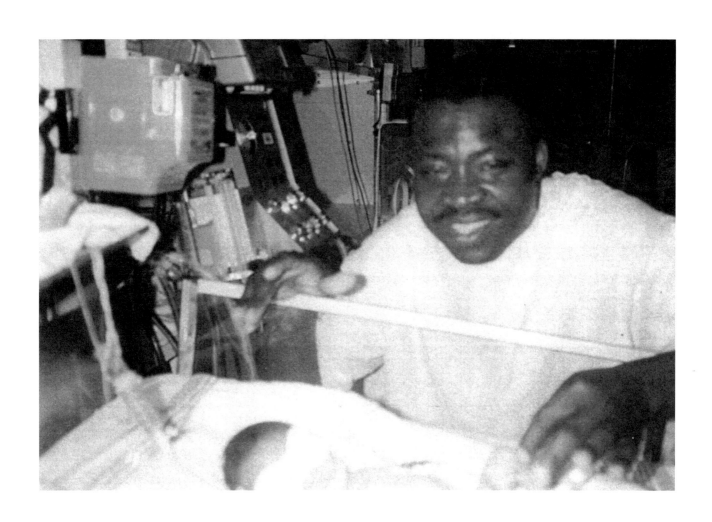

CHAPTER 15
FIBROIDS: 3/10/1997

HIGH RISK PREGNANCY WITH DEGENERATIVE FIBROSIS:

Operative Finding: The uterus was noted to have a large left cornual angle fibroid. Three days after the delivery I ran into the doctor/surgeon on a wheelchair ride to the NICU to see my son for the first time. He was happy to see me and wondered what happened to me. I asked him if I had died during surgery? He implied that I had not died. He also said that I was very anxious during the procedure. In speaking with him, it was noted that he saw the fibroid and said he was happy that it was not covering the baby. It was a large cornual shaped fibroid that could have caused problems during surgery. I then asked why it was not taken out? He said, "*It couldn't be taken out because it may have caused too much bleeding.*"

Recently, after hearing so much about bleeding and after care. I asked my sister, (Karin), now mother of four, what was to be expected during bleeding after delivery? She said, '*they warn you about blood clots, size and to notify someone immediately if it becomes excessive.*' Also, with all the talk about UTERINE FIBROIDS in the news I thought why not utilize this space and place the MAYO CLINIC information below for easy reference:

Fibroids: The 411 - CARE About Fibroids

Uterine Fibroids: A Common But Rarely Discussed Condition. On behalf of the many women now suffering in silence, CARE About Fibroids is dedicated to taking uterine fibroids out of the shadows. This starts by raising awareness of this medical condition so women will recognize the signs and symptoms, know the risk factors, and know how to discuss ...

Uterine Fibroids: A Common But Rarely Discussed Condition

On behalf of the many women now suffering in silence, CARE About Fibroids is dedicated to taking uterine fibroids out of the shadows. This starts by raising awareness of this medical condition so women will recognize the signs and symptoms, know the risk factors, and know how to discuss fibroids with their gynecologist, family doctor, and other health care professionals. CARE About Fibroids believes that knowledge and awareness will help more women get an earlier diagnosis of uterine fibroids and choose an appropriate treatment that reflects their health situation.

Fibroids: The 411. CARE About Fibroids. (n.d.). http://www.careaboutfibroids.org/411.html

It's Not Normal: Black Women, Stop Suffering From Fibroids

Women may not recognize that they have a problem for months or years, resulting in a delay in treatment, and physical, economic, and emotional costs.

By HealthyWomen EditorsApr 02, 2019

Editors, H. (2022, June 22). It's not normal: Black women, stop suffering from fibroids. HealthyWomen. https://www.healthywomen.org/content/article/its-not-normal-black-women-stop-suffering-fibroids

CHAPTER 16
SENT HOME WITHOUT MEDS: 3/12/1997

It **just** hit me that on March 12, 1997, I was discharged from the hospital and went home without ever having held my baby. I wasn't allowed to hold him until I could sit down in one of those old ass rocking chairs. The seat was too low for anyone's comfort. Just as I was about to leave for discharge, I was given an intensive two-hour orientation and instruction on how to do infant CPR and care. The orientation room was small and was very warm/hot. With my pressure being up and other conditions, I felt really faint. What made it worse, I was completely following along with an intensity that I really didn't have in me.

The potholes in the streets in the city of buffalo were absolutely horrendous and made the drive home pretty painful. I couldn't sit down, my body was tense and rigid in the car. By the time we made it home my body was in complete distress. I couldn't physically relax my body enough to sit down, sit back nor lean on the sofa. I somehow made my way up the stairs to the bedroom where I stayed until my appointment that Friday.

While at home I noticed that when I would urinate my entire bladder felt like it would dislodge momentarily and then return to its original state. As the days went on, I remembered the last couple of days before I left the hospital. Once they took the catheter out, I had all the patterns of a urinary tract infection. After I settled in, I found copies of the hospital brochure explaining what a urinary tract infection consisted of. I was definitely infected according to what I was going through. I took the liberty of trying to solve the problem myself by guzzling down a couple gallons of cranberry juice and lots of water. Fortunately, I had a scheduled blood pressure check in two days, Friday, March 14, 1997, and would be going back to the hospital. The blood work from my appointment in fact confirmed a urinary tract infection. (The infection had pretty much cleared up due to guzzling down cranberry juice and water). Also, at that appointment, it was discovered that my blood pressure was SKY HIGH.

They were in the process of calling the ambulance to send me over to Buffalo General Hospital because Children's Hospital did not treat High Blood Pressure outside of Maternity admission. I didn't want to go, I wanted to go to the NICU to see my baby. Especially after receiving a call that I needed to come and see my baby because sometimes social services may take it.. Of course, I was afraid and didn't want them to take my baby.

To make this possible, someone from the pharmacy ran across the street to Rite Aid and purchased some high blood pressure meds. They stuck two dissolving pills, one at a time, under my tongue. I then asked, "*Why was my body jerking*?" The nurse responded that '*I was trying to go into convulsions?!*'

The symptoms are, if you have hypertension eclampsia: you can have seizures, lapse into a coma and die. To think, they had the incompetent audacity to send me home without any blood pressure meds. Nothing for my bladder infection or information regarding blood clots. Nor did I receive a script for prenatal vitamins just told that I could buy them over the counter. The night before I was discharged from the hospital my reflexes were off the chain. To the point where I had an uncontrollable jerking to my body. (It's called hyper-reflexes, something I'm currently **aware** of.) I was afraid to be left alone, so Uzo stayed the night with me. My reflexes were jerking so hard that I thought I was going to fall out of the bed. I had fevers and chills out of nowhere. I couldn't get warm. They bought me warm blankets, but I was still cold. It wasn't until the catheter was taken out that my blood flow started. (The nurse had implied upon my arrival back to my 5th floor original room, '*that I was the cleanest patient that she ever had because there was no bleeding.*') However, once it started, I remember bleeding clots. I would put down bed pads on the floor in the bathroom to dispose of my personal hygiene products, which were loaded with blood. Uzo would wrap everything up and dispose of it when he would visit. Once or twice, I would call the nurse in to help because I couldn't bend or stoop low enough to handle it myself. Only recently after hearing so much in the news about bleeding, hemorrhaging and blood clots, I again, then asked my sister what was the protocol after a delivery. She informed me that she was told, '*if any blood clots were formed bigger than the size of a quarter to notify someone immediately.*' This was my first time ever hearing of such a warning. Although some patients' mortality may have resulted in not being warned, what about the sheer numbers that died from simply not being listened to?! Either way, more education and knowledge on all levels is critical.

Going to the bathroom was the worst for me. I would struggle over to the toilet, lean my left shoulder and head on to the wall for support with slightly bent knees and slide down the wall while hovering over the toilet, then the urine would pour out. I would make it to the bathroom just in time every time. That was the easy part. The really, really hard part was how I got there! First, I had to be barefooted on the tile floor. Then turn my body sideways in the direction I was headed. That was to the bathroom. Remember, I was in a physically rigid posture without any flexibility in my hip flexor region. While leaning forward and keeping floor contact with slightly bent knees, I would scrunch my toes, really, really fast, (that gave me momentum) and wiggle the heels and ball of my feet from side to side. *Scrunch, scrunch, wiggle, wiggle; scrunch, scrunch; wiggle, wiggle; scrunch, scrunch, wiggle, wiggle*. Repeatedly, all the way to the toilet. Again, making it just in time, every time. And, still there was something worse than that, which was: not having use of my hip flexors, climbing in and out of bed was already difficult because my feet could not reach the floor from the bed which remained in an inclined position.

Once the catheter had been removed, my bladder would fill and I needed to urinate non stop, which I did. So, I would pump the Demerol to help ease the pain so that I wouldn't feel the pain as much. Then, I would stay in bed and nod for a while, never knowing why.

MR#:   002149928
Name: CHILLIS, ELEANORE
DOB: 06/08/56
Date of Admission: 02/27/97
Date of Discharge: 03/12/97

Dict: ███████-Di████, M.D.
ETD/12950
6777

Dictated: 03/12/97
Transcribed: 03/13/97

cc: ███████ Women's Clinic
    ███████-Di████ M.D.-Variety 5

DISCHARGE SUMMARY

ATTENDING PHYSICIAN: █████████████ M.D.

ADMISSION DIAGNOSIS:
1.   Intrauterine pregnancy at 31 and 1/7 weeks gestation.
2.   Mild preeclampsia.
3.   Degenerating uterine fibroids.
4.   ████████████████
5.   Intrauterine growth retardation.
6.   Advanced maternal age.
7.   Desiring permanent surgical sterilization.

DISCHARGE DIAGNOSIS:
1.   Status post delivery of a viable male infant by primary low-flap transverse
        cesarean section.
2.   Status post bilateral tubal ligation by modified Pomeroy.
3.   Status post severe preeclampsia on magnesium.
4.   Elevated blood pressures.

HISTORY OF PRESENT ILLNESS: The patient is a 40-year-old black female G1, P0,
with an LMP of 7/25/96 and EDC of 4/27/97 by a 12 week ultrasound who presented
to Children's labor and delivery at 31 and 1/7 weeks gestation complaining of a
headache, blurry vision, and lower extremity swelling. The patient stated that
she had a history of three degenerating fibroids and had been in excruciating
pain throughout the day despite Tylenol with codeine. The patient denied any
history of hypertension.

Prenatal labs: ███████ Rubella immune, VDRL nonreactive, hepatitis B
surface antigen negative, ████████████

PAST MEDICAL HISTORY: ████████████, hypertension denied.

PAST SURGICAL HISTORY: Denied.

ALLERGIES: No known drug allergies.

MEDICATIONS: Prenatal vitamins, Tylenol with codeine.

FAMILY HISTORY: Denied.

SOCIAL HISTORY: Quit smoking four years prior to presentation. She denied any
tobacco or alcohol use.

PAST GYN HISTORY: She denied any sexually transmitted diseases.

CONTINUED. . .

MR#: 002149928
Name: CHILLIS, ELEANORE

PHYSICAL EXAMINATION: On physical examination she was found to have a blood pressure of 136/82. Her cervix was found to be fingertip, thick, and high. Cervical cultures were not done because the patient could not tolerate a speculum exam. On the monitor the fetus was found to have a heart rate in the 130's to 140's with average variability and accelerations. No uterine contractions were noted. On the ultrasound a single vertex fetus was noted with an AUA of 28 and 1/7 weeks, estimated fetal weight of 1,104 grams. AFI was 10.1 cm and a posterior placenta with a BPP of 8/10.

HOSPITAL COURSE AND TREATMENT: Thus the patient was admitted at 31 and 1/7 weeks gestation in order to rule out preeclampsia. She has a history of degenerating fibroids with pain, desires a postpartum tubal. She is a ▒▒▒▒ with IUGR, advanced maternal age, and an elevated maternal serum alpha fetoprotein of 5.5 MOM. She refused amnio in the past. The patient's 24-hour urine showed a protein excretion of 522 mg over 24 hours. CBC and SMA-18 were within normal limits except for a uric acid of 6.9. Platelets were normal at 211. The patient's prenatal course was without complications. She was monitored carefully up on V5, received betamethasone. Once during her hospitalization on 3/4/97 the patient was transferred down to V3 because of regular uterine contractions that were very painful. These contractions petered-out and the patient's cervix did not change, thus she was sent back up to V5 for continued observation of fetal well being and mild preeclampsia. On the 6th the patient's blood pressures became elevated up to 164/105. She was at this point dipping +3 proteinuria whereas compared to her baseline of +1 to +2. Her deep tendon reflexes were increased at 3+ and she was found to have 1-2 beats of clonus. Thus, the patient was transferred again down to V3 on the 6th for severe preeclampsia demonstrated by an increase in blood pressure, increase in edema, increase in proteinuria, and hyperreflexia. That morning the patient had undergone an amnio for lung maturity which was found to be immature at 22. The patient was started on magnesium sulfate, received a second dose of her two runs of betamethasone and then on the 8th underwent a primary low-flap transverse cesarean section with bilateral tubal ligation with a delivery of a viable male infant, Apgars of 6 at one minute, 8 at five minutes with a weight of 3 lb. 4 oz., 1,476 grams, pH of 7.23, base excess of -1 and hemoglobin of 14.9. The patient was continued on magnesium sulfate for another 24 hours and then on the 5th was sent up to the floor. Although her blood pressures initially came down during her postpartum course, it was noted that the patient's blood pressures continued to be high with a range of 120 to 180/74 to 105. On postpartum day four, on March 12th, the patient was discharged to home.

DISCHARGE: The patient was discharged on 3/12/97 to home with a prescription for Tylenol and Codeine #3 and followup in four weeks in the Women's Clinic and in two days on Friday in the clinic for a blood pressure check. She is also to followup with physical therapy for continued outpatient rehab and preeclampsia precautions were reviewed with the patient.

OBSTETRICAL AND SHORT-STAY GYN

DISCHARGE SUMMARY

DISCHARGE DATE: 3/12/97

```
MR 2 14 99 28        16C
CHILLIS, ELEANORE ████████, M.D.
SEX: F
PA# 4704856   DOB: 06/08/56
                          ADM:02/27/97
```

Addressograph

ADMISSION DIAGNOSIS: [ ] IUP/Labor   [X] Pregnancy

[ ] Fertility   [ ] DUB

Other: _Preterm pregnancy & Intrauterine growth retard_
Oligohydramnios, mild preeclampsia

PROCEDURE(S):

[ ] Spontaneous Vaginal   [ ] Operative Vaginal   [ ] D&C   [ ] Breast Biopsy
    Delivery   Delivery

[X] C-Section   [ ] ETP   [ ] Tubal   [ ] Diagnostic
                                                      Ligation   Laparoscopy

Other: _Bilat tubal ligation_

DISCHARGE DIAGNOSIS: [X] IUP Delivered   [ ] IUP Undelivered

Other: _None_

MEDICATIONS: _T+C #3_

CONDITION ON DISCHARGE: _Stable_

DISCHARGE INSTRUCTIONS: [ ] Postpartum   [X] Post C-Section

POSTOP: [ ] Tubal   [ ] D&C   [ ] Diagnostic Lap   [ ] Breast Biopsy

Other: _____

FOLLOW-UP: _4-6 wks clinic, F/u Friday 3/14 for BP √ in clinic_
_F/u c̄ P.T._

████████████████   3/12/97
M.D. Signature   Date

5/91

56

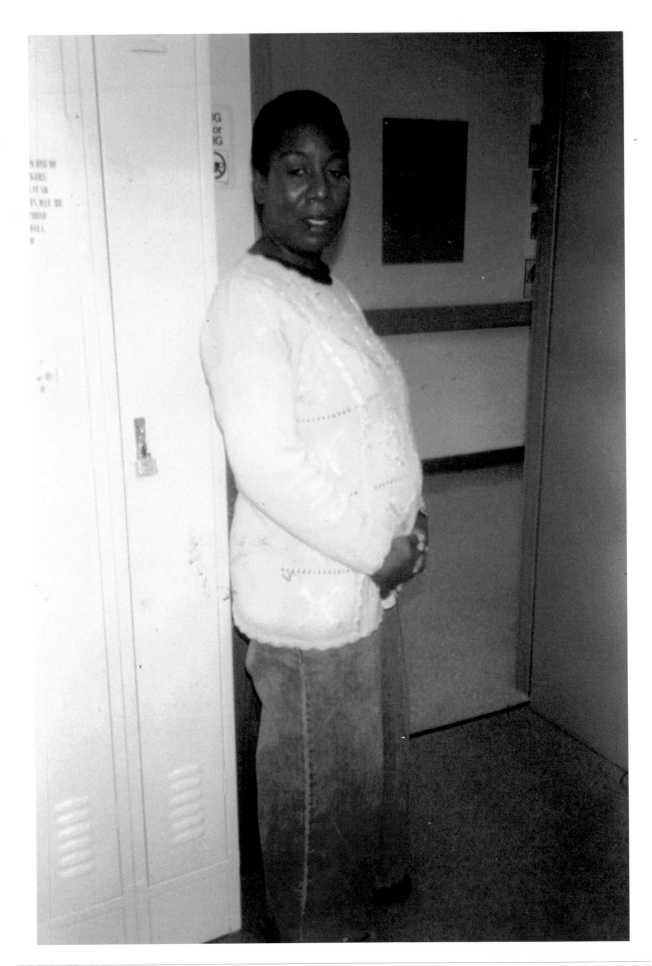

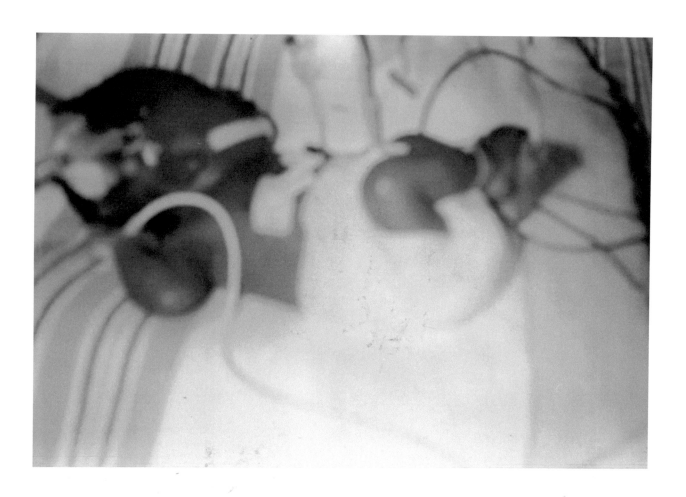

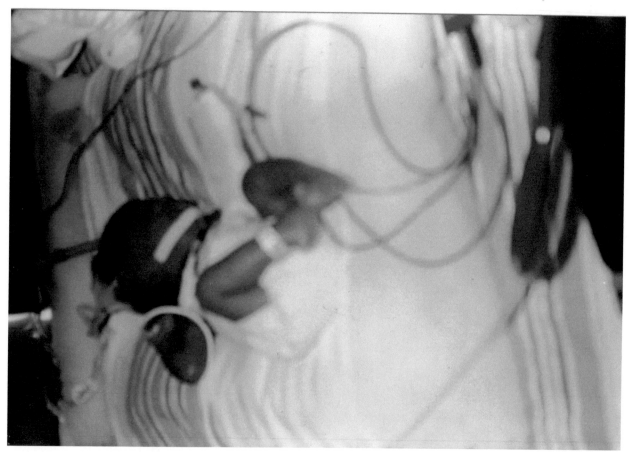

SENT HOME WITHOUT MEDS: 3/12/1997

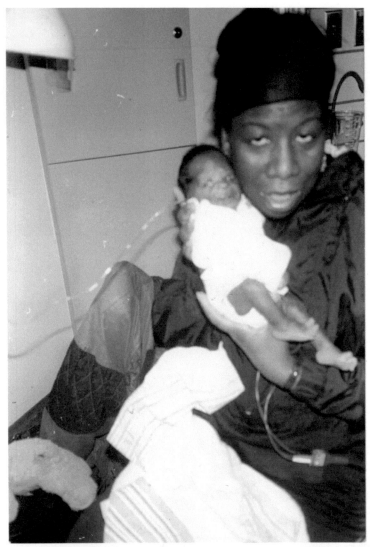

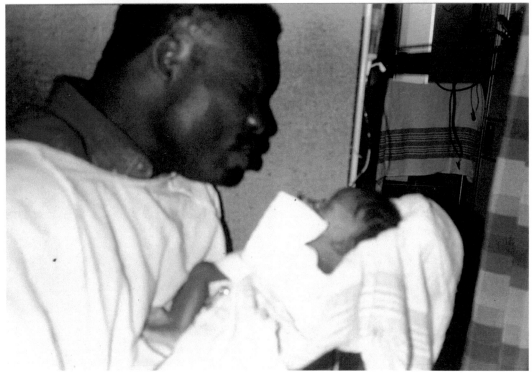

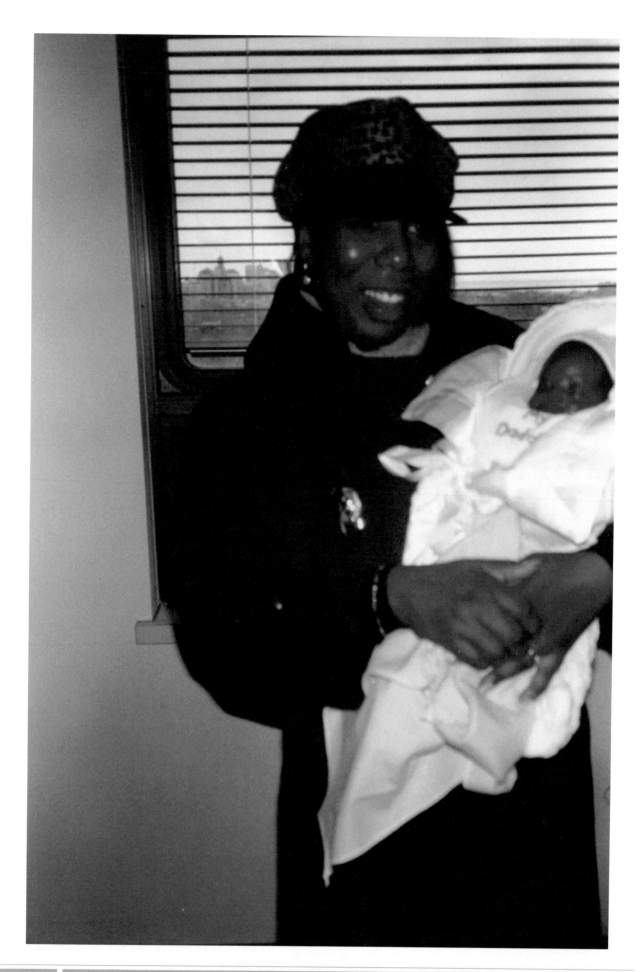

SENT HOME WITHOUT MEDS: 3/12/1997

CHAPTER 17
LEARNING TO WALK AGAIN: 3/15/1997 - 6/15/1997

The General Observation was the loss of use of my Hip Flexors with little mobility and no flexibility, a painful condition that progressively progressed from the onset of my pregnancy and its entirety. This condition was never properly addressed; although, there was some concern of my legs deconditioning. It wasn't until I was being discharged from the hospital that I asked about my condition and the fact that I couldn't walk when I was admitted to the hospital and now that I've had surgery I really couldn't walk, correctly. I thought this was something that would have been addressed during my stay/delivery. Then, at that time, a therapist was called to assess my condition.

Second position turnout is a Russian Ballet Dance Position:

I had all of the bed pillows on the 5th floor, on my bed, because I couldn't lie flat, unaware that I had a hip problem. The hip flexor did not work, nor did I know what or how it connected to my inability to walk, sit or lie down flat. All I knew is that it was very difficult to stand up from a seated position or sit down from a standing position; getting in and out of a car where I needed assistance because I couldn't relax my rigid posture.

Before surgery, I had to throw my legs in order to walk. While standing from a seated position and to keep from falling, I would straddle my legs wide, with my feet spread apart in order to balance and distribute my body weight evenly over my legs, with both hands pressing along my thighs and in order to stand upright. And, from there with feet pronated and rolled inwards, while flat footed I slowly scooted them inwards in order to walk. From the hips down I was rotated with a *turned out* 2nd position in ballet, with my feet pronated and rolled inwards. After surgery, I was in a contracted fifth position turnout, i.e., 90 degrees from the hips. This contracted position was never released until I went to therapy to learn to walk correctly again. My best guess is 6 - 8 weeks or 3 months. Once baby Kelechi was discharged from the hospital my mom would come to babysit him while I continued my weekly therapy sessions. Because my feet had been rotated outwards from the hips down the length of my legs for so long, I had to first learn how to turn my feet straight and focused on walking forward.

It was a struggle, but I got through it. Yet through it all, I couldn't imagine this TRUTH that had actually happened to me. No one seemed concerned, let alone listened to me. What a nightmare!

Last, but not least, I wasn't going to mention what had happened the night or two before my discharge; but a nurse bought my meds for me, (Tylenol with codeine) for pain. However, because I've never liked taking meds, I told the nurse that I would like to skip my scheduled round of Tylenol's. At that time, she became really mad and insisted that I had to take it. I then took the pill from her and threw it under the bed where it remained until I left for home. Note, she came back later to apologize. Yet, I was sent home with a high blood pressure of 180/105 without a prescription. *Hmm!*

CHAPTER 18

INFANT MORBIDITY, MORTALITY OR SIDS: 4/6/1997 - 4/1998 (VOLUME #2)

Why did they move him out of the NICUa so soon? And, onto the 2nd stage NICUb, then Premie-land and was discharged within 29 days of his birth, with a breathing problem. I dictated breathing difficulties as soon as he arrived home from the Hospital. Kelechi would stop breathing 15 seconds at a time every time he slept. Why did the NICU not detect this? It was never mentioned to me as they always had noted all other infant conditions.

Such as, when he had something called neck (a condition when the baby is not digesting feed through the feeding tube in his mouth; and how they really didn't want to shave his/Kelechi's beautiful hair to feed nutrients through a feeding tube in the right temple in his head).

Previously as a Marketing Coordinator and Production Assistant for over $650,000 worth of Financial Banking products where I also Tracked & Reported over 3,500 million piece mailings as a Fulfillment Analyst & Marketing Coordinator of Direct Response Marketing. I've learned to become very intuitive and attuned to details.

And as I observed those conditions in my son's breathing pattern, I started tracking and logging each episode onto my 1997 and 1998 wall calendar. The patterns of noisy sounds, rhythms, and descriptions of his struggles to breathe. Everything, from a rubber band vibrating to a banjo playing, etc., yet not one time was he ever snoring. The sound was very distinctive and destructive. Of course, I almost never slept, because I was always writing, and jarring him awake.

It was a good thing, because at that time, I was not working, in addition to being a baby hogger (loving to hold babies). So, I held him a lot. He never liked laying across my lap which I found quite alarming because he was a very calm, quiet and happy baby. Other, than his noisy breathing, not snoring…, two different things. So, to the point, I didn't then and don't know now, what his crying pattern sounds like, because there wasn't much crying. However, I can even tell you about the handful of times he did cry. He was a very content baby whose needs were always met.

The end result of it all was for 13 months or about 371 days KELECHI would stop breathing for 15 seconds EVERY time he slept. That's 371 days, up to a number of times/minutes/hours he slept-daily. (*Go figure*!). An infant's struggle to breathe for approximately 371 days… story continues in Volume 2… (INFANT MORBIDITY, MORTALITY OR SIDS)

SPECIAL THANKS

- Uncle Wardell & Aunt Glorine Linder who held all of our families in Buffalo together.
- Uzo Ihenko, Ph.D, is always there and supportive, never skipping or missing a beat. Matter of fact, let me tell y'all something, y'all ready know, about Uzo…. Hands down, Uzo works harder than any and everybody I know and gets the job done every time. He is a giver of time and resources and makes it happen! Uzo1 is your connection to the world and the finder of all things. If it exists on this earth, he will get it and If it doesn't exist, he'll let you know that it can't be found. I call him "the Energizer Bunny that takes a licking and keeps on ticking!"
- Sop Ihenko, a Science Professor in Biology and Integrated Science and final book editor. Sop Kelechi's Aunt kept the family meals coming relentlessly with praise and encouragement in my efforts while writing this book.
- Kelechi was a good baby and always waited patiently for my daily visit to the hospital NICU. It was because of him, I am writing this book.
- James & Maureen Wright opened their home to me upon my arrival in California; Sondra & Lish Gordon, Michelle Samuel & Joe Davis, California friends; Late District Attorney Estella Dooley for giving me my 1st California job; Mary Comer Fong for being a very special friend & supportive co-worker, California; Ethal Jean Wright, Wrightsville Ga. Historian
- Stacey Wirth a true and trusted friend who is always there.
- Sheila L. Brown, SLB Academy
- Bernie Taylor, Brown & Taylor Associates, Literary Agent
- Pam James, MA, MS and (CEO, LifeSource System, Inc.) business partner and book foreward writer
- Ashley Chamberlain, MBA was committed and trusted with my first edits while studying for a BS RN degree in nursing.
- Kendra Lawrence, LPN today that helped nurse me back to health at 2 years old & researched the operative procedure & medical word definitions for this writing.
- Karin is always cooking something & the caregiver of my mother during her sickness & elder years. She did for my mother what I wasn't free to do.
- Sharon is a hard worker and helped out with my mom to the end.
- Keenan who always planted a daily kiss onto moms cheek and for being the strong arm to help Karin and Kendra move her about.
- Margo Chillis-Harber a dedicated sister-in-law
- William (Mann) for taking on the role of a strong family man who has recently transcended
- Willie Chillis is supportive and was always being pulled in many directions to do a job for one of his many (8) sisters.
- Sierra is always very helpful, reliable and a very caring person
- Joyce holding strong to her beliefs and the community needs of others
- Janet a strong will and impressive voice for cultural change

- Judy was my "Sister Mary" growing up and a dedicated mother raising her 4 daughters
- Kevin our #1 family sports star and world traveler
- Sabrina for being there and her commitment to Uncle William
- Myself for listening and knowing how to use my GOD given knowledge, Yeah that's me!

IN REMEMBRANCE OF

Grandmother, Clara (Ball) Wright
Father, Ulysese Chillis
Mother, Hazel Chillis
Uncle, William Wright
Brother, William Chillis
Sister, Margaret Chillis
Sister, Suzanna Chillis
Sister-in-Law, Alexandra Kijonek
Nephew, William (Mann)
Nephew, Sam (Smokie)
Nephew, Marvin (Lumpy)
Nephew, Donnie
Nephew, Lonnie (Boo)
Great Great Nephew, Shawn
Great Great Niece, Cianna
First Cousin, Geraldine Dubose
First Cousin, Jerry Linder
Third Cousin, Keyshawn
Family, Friend Ms Boone
Family, Friend Mr. James

5/14/2022 and the Jefferson Ave 10, Buffalo, NY, Tops MASSACRE

Celestine Chaney
Roberta A. Drury
Andre Mackneil
Katherine Massey
Margus D. Morrison
Deacon Heyward Patterson
Aaron Salter
Geraldine Talley
Ruth Whitfield
Pearly Young

OPERATIVE REPORT MEDICAL TERMS

NOTE: (From Medical Report listed in order of events)

INTRA-UTERINE PREGNANCY

INTRA-UTERINE GROWTH RESTRICTION (IUGR)

ECLAMPSIA

SEVERE ECLAMPSIA

SEVERE PRE-ECLAMPSIA

OLIGOHYDRAMNIOS

DEGENERATING FIBROIDS

DORSAL SUPINE POSITION

C-SECTION

CESAREAN

EPIDURAL ANESTHESIA

IV SEDATION

DEMEROL

TORADOL

PERIANTH

POMERY

CORNUAL PANGLE FIBROID

FIBROID

PFANNENSTIEL

DISSECTED

RECTUS MUSCLES

PERITONEAL

RECTUS MUSCLES

PERITONEAL

PERITONEUM

VESICOUTERINE PERITONEUM

BLADDER FLAP

ATRAUMATICALLY

AMNION NODOSUM

0 MONOCRYL

UTERINE INCISION

0 VICRYL

HEMOSTASIS

FALLOPIAN TUBE

POMEROY

0 CHROMIC SUTURE

AVASCULAR SECTION

FOLEY CATHETER

POSTPARTUM WARD

IV SEDATION CONTINUED

PRE-ECLAMPSIE

MAGNESIUM SULFATE

OPERATIVE REPORT MEDICAL TERMS & DEFINITIONS

Note: (From Operative Report listed in order of events)

INTRA-UTERINE PREGNANCY - is a medical condition in which a fertilized sac is implanted in the uterus

IUGR - refers to when a baby has poor growth in the womb

ECLAMPSIA - is severe hypertension

SEVERE PRE-ECLAMPSIA - new onset of hypertension typically around the 20th week of pregnancy

OLIGOHYDRAMNIOS - is when there is too little amniotic fluid

FIBROID DEGENERATION - is when a FIBROID stops receiving enough nutrients from its blood supply

SUPINE - this position consumes a patient to lie flat on their back, face and abdomen facing upward

EPIDURAL ANESTHESIA - is an injection that is placed into the space between the wall of the spinal canal and the covering of the spinal cord

C-SECTION - same as Cesarean

CESAREAN - Cesarean section, also known as C-section or cesarean delivery, is the surgical procedure by which one or more babies are delivered through an incision in the mother's abdomen

IV SEDATION - is a conscious sedation to help you relax during a procedure

DEMEROL - is used to treat moderate to severe pain (opioid)

TORADOL - Toradol - is a short term to reduce pain in adults. Typically used before or after medical procedures and after surgery (NSAID)

POMEROY - removal/resection of the fallopian tube. Often times part of the tube is tied around the segment

CORNUAL PANGLE FIBROID - in the upper corner of the uterus (cornual region) can occasionally obstruct fallopian tubes and can be a cause of tubal factor subfertility. Similarly, very large fibroids and an enlarged uterine cavity be a cause of not getting pregnant

FIBROID - are muscular tumors that grow in the wall of the uterus (womb)

PFANNENSTIEL - a transverse lower abdominal incision that is made superior to the pubic ridge

DISSECTED - to cut or separate tissue into pieces

RECTUS ABDOMINIS - makes up the top layer of your abdominal muscles

PERITONEUM - tissue that lines the abdominal wall and pelvis (parietal layer)

VESICOUTERINE POUCH - is a fold of the peritoneum from the bladder to the body of the uterus in the female

BLADDER FLAP - is created by superficially incising and dissecting the peritoneal lining to separate the urinary bladder from the lower uterine segment

ATRAUMATICALLY - is designed to minimize tissue damage; not causing injury or trauma

AMNION NODOSUM - is commonly regarded as a placental hallmark of severe and prolonged oligohydramnios

MONOCRYL SUTURES - are indicated for use in several soft tissue and/or where an absorbable material is indicated

UTERINE INCISION - is a surgical procedure in which there is an incision is made in the mothers abdomen and uterus

VICRYL - is an absorbable, synthetic, usually braided suture. It is indicated for use in general soft tissue approximation and/or ligation, including ophthalmic procedures, but not cardiovascular or neurological tissues

HEMOSTASIS - is a process that stops or arrest bleeding

FALLOPIAN TUBE - one of the two fallopian tubes that carry the egg from the ovary to the uterus

CHROMIC SUTURE - dissolvable biological suture material

MONOCRYL SUTURES - are indicated for use in several soft tissue and/or where an absorbable material is indicate

POMEROY - Pomeroy - removal/resection of the fallopian tube. Often times part of the tube is tied around the segment

AVASCULAR SECTION - is a condition in which there is a loss of blood flow to the bone tissue, which causes the bone to die

FOLEY CATHETER - Foley is a small flexible rubber or plastic tube that is placed into the bladder to assist in the collection and drainage of urine for those who have medical conditions affecting their urinary tract

BETAMETHASONE - is a highly potent steroid that prevents the release of substance in the body that causes inflammation and also used for many other medical problems

MAGNESIUM SULFATE - is used to treat to prevent seizures seizures in women with preeclampsia

OPERATIVE REPORT MEDICAL TERMS & PROCEDURES DURING C-SECTION

Note: (From Medical Report listed in order of events)

OLIGOHYDRAMNIOS - low amniotic fluid

SUPINE POSITION - lying flat on a slightly angled operating

PERIANTH - all the structures surrounding the reproductive

EPIDURAL ANESTHESIA - used during delivery

C-SECTION - same as a Cesarean

CESAREAN - Cesarean section, also known as C-section or Cesarean delivery, is the surgical procedure by which one or more babies are delivered through an incision in the mother's abdomen

PFANNENSTIEL - scalpel incision in skin through fascia/fascial elevated

SCALPEL - used to make incisions

MAYO SCISSORS - fascial incision extended bilaterally with the scissors

KOCHER CLAMPS - use to grasped the Fascial

DISSECTED - the fascial incision was elevated and both sharply and bluntly dissected both superiorly and inferiorly from the rectus muscles

RECTUS MUSCLES - separated in midline (incision)

PERITONEUM - was tented up and entered bluntly and extended

IV SEDATION - additional sedation was given

PERITONEAL INCISION - was extended superiorly and inferiorly

BLADDER BLADE - was inserted

VESICOUTERINE PERITONEUM - grasped with the pickups & entered sharply with the metzenbaum scissors

METZENBAUM SCISSORS - were used for the Vesicouterine Peritoneum

BLADDER FLAP - incision extended laterally creating the Bladder Flap & restricted downward using the bladder blade

CORNUAL ANGLE FIBROID - located on the left side of Uterines

FIBROID - large Fibroid was not covering the infant during delivery

ATRAUMATICALLY - infants head and body delivered atraumatically

PLACENTA - preterm placenta with three infarcts

UTERINE - incision repaired in a running locking fashion in a single larger with O Monocryl with noted small blood vessel at right angle of the uterine incision

HEMOSTASIS - good Hemostasis achieved with three figure-of-eight sutures using O Vicryl

POMEROY - tubal ligation modified

AMNION NODOSUM - severe prolonged placental Oligohydraminos

FOLEY CATHETER - inserted

MAGNESIUM SULFATE - an additional 24 hours of IV treatment

PREGNANCY RELATED TERMS

Proteinuria - pre-eclampsia is a complication of pregnancy. With preeclampsia, you might have high blood pressure, high levels of protein in urine that indicate kidney damage (proteinuria), or other signs of organ damage. Pre-eclampsia usually begins after 20 weeks of pregnancy in women whose blood pressure had previously been in the standard range.

Left untreated, pre-eclampsia can lead to serious - even fatal - complications for both the mother and baby.

Early delivery of the baby is often recommended. The timing of delivery depends on how severe the pre-eclampsia is and how many weeks pregnant you are.

Before delivery, preeclampsia treatment includes careful monitoring and medications to lower blood pressure and manage complications.

Per-eclampsia may develop after delivery of a baby, a condition known as postpartum preeclampsia.

Mayo Foundation for Medical Education and Research. (2022, April 15). Pre-eclampsia. Mayo Clinic. https://www.mayoclinic.org/diseases-conditions/preeclampsia/symptoms-causes/syc-20355745

Gestational proteinuria - is a subset of isolated proteinuria which is defined as proteinuria with onset after 20 weeks in the absence of hypertension [22].

Since gestational proteinuria often progresses to preeclampsia, it is a retrospective diagnosis that may only be made postpartum if preeclampsia does not develop.

Mayo Foundation for Medical Education and Research. (2022, April 15). Gestational proteinuria Preeclampsia . Mayo Clinic. https://www.mayoclinic.org/diseases-conditions/preeclampsia/symptoms-causes/syc-20355745

Vasculitis - Pregnancy and vasculitis: a systematic review of the literature Primary systemic vasculitis are uncommon diseases that may affect young women in their childbearing age. To date, patients affected with primary systemic vasculitis are often diagnosed and treated earlier than in the past, due to improvement in diagnostic skills and a larger availability of effective drugs.

Gatto M;Iaccarino L;Canova M;Zen M;Nalotto L;Ramonda R;Punzi L;Doria A; (n.d.). Pregnancy and vasculitis: A systematic review of the literature. Autoimmunity reviews. https://pubmed.ncbi.nlm.nih.gov/22155197/

Author links open overlay panelMariele Gatto, AbstractPrimary systemic vasculitis are uncommon diseases that may affect young women in their childbearing age. To date, Ishikawa, K., Wong, V. C. W., Sharma, B. K., Grewal, K., Rocha, M. P., Hampl, J. C., Herrema, I., Winn, H. N., Chua, S., Askie, L. M., Sibai, B., Nagey, D. A., Owen, J., Aya, A. G., Dayoan, E. S., Bessias, N., M'Rad, S., … Graca, L. M. (2011, December 3). Pregnancy and vasculitis: A systematic review of the literature. Autoimmunity Reviews. https://www.sciencedirect.com/science/article/abs/pii/S156899721100293X

Thrombosis - is a blood clot within blood vessels that limits the flow of blood. Acute venous and arterial thromboses are the most common cause of death in developed countries. The mortality rate varies with the location and acuity of thrombosis.

professional, C. C. medical. (n.d.-d). Thrombosis: What you need to know. Cleveland Clinic. https://my.clevelandclinic.org/health/diseases/22242-thrombosis

Thrombosis is the medical term for when a blood clot, or "thrombus," forms a blockage inside a blood vessel. The thrombus limits or blocks blood flow to the parts of the body that the vessel usually supplies, causing symptoms in those areas.

MediLexicon International. (n.d.-a). Thrombosis: Types, symptoms, treatment, and more. Medical News Today. https://www.medicalnewstoday.com/articles/thrombosis

Ischemia of the Placenta - Pre-eclampsia, intre-uterine growth restriction, and placental abruption are serious obstetrical complications that constitute the syndrome of ischemic placental disease and account for a disproportionate degree of perinatal morbidity and mortality.

AM;, A. C. (n.d.). Ischemic placental disease and risks of perinatal mortality and morbidity and neurodevelopmental outcomes. Seminars in perinatology. https://pubmed.ncbi.nlm.nih.gov/24836827/

Associate with RA and SEL

Rheumatoid arthritis, or RA, is an autoimmune and inflammatory disease, which means that your immune system attacks healthy cells in your body by mistake, causing inflammation (painful swelling) in the affected parts of the body. RA mainly attacks the joints, usually many joints at once. RA commonly affects joints in the hands, wrists, and knees.

Centers for Disease Control and Prevention. (2020, July 27). Rheumatoid arthritis (RA). Centers for Disease Control and Prevention. https://www.cdc.gov/arthritis/basics/rheumatoid-arthritis.html

Systemic lupus erythematosus (SLE), is the most common type of lupus. SLE is an autoimmune disease in which the immune system attacks its own tissues, causing widespread inflammation and tissue damage in the affected organs. It can affect the joints, skin, brain, lungs, kidneys, and blood vessels. There is no cure for lupus, but medical interventions and lifestyle changes can help control it.

Centers for Disease Control and Prevention. (2022, July 5). Systemic lupus erythematosus (SLE). Centers for Disease Control and Prevention. https://www.cdc.gov/lupus/facts/detailed.html

Autoimmune Disorders - The exact cause of autoimmune disorders is unknown. One theory is that some microorganisms (such as bacteria or viruses) or drugs may trigger changes that confuse the immune system. This may happen more often in people who have genes that make them more prone to autoimmune disorders.

U.S. National Library of Medicine. (n.d.). Autoimmune disorders: Medlineplus medical encyclopedia. MedlinePlus. https://medlineplus.gov/ency/article/000816.htm

Autoimmune Disease - Autoimmune diseases are a case of mistaken identity in which the body's immune system, which ordinarily attacks intruders like viruses and bacteria, attacks itself. There are more than 100 different autoimmune diseases, some of which involve a single organ (e.g. Hashimoto's thyroiditis) and others that attack nearly any organ or tissue (e.g. lupus).

Early symptoms, such as fatigue and joint pain, mimic those of other medical conditions, making diagnosis challenging. These conditions can be temporary or, more commonly, lifelong. They're sometimes referred to as "invisible disabilities," since people may not appear outwardly ill despite dealing with significant issues.

Shomon, M. (n.d.). Know the symptoms of some common autoimmune conditions. Verywell Health. https://www.verywellhealth.com/autoimmune-disease-symptoms-3232847

Thrombus vs Embolus - thrombosis is when a blood clot, or thrombus, forms in a blood vessel. An embolus is when a clot, fat, air bubble, or other feature travels through blood vessels, with a risk of lodging elsewhere. Both can block blood flow and increase the risk of a heart attack or stroke.

MediLexicon International. (n.d.-b). Thrombosis vs. embolism: Differences, symptoms, and more. Medical News Today. https://www.medicalnewstoday.com/articles/thrombosis-vs-embolism

Placenta - 1 a flattened circular organ in the uterus of pregnant eutherian mammals, nourishing and maintaining the fetus through the umbilical cord.

The placenta consists of vascular tissue in which oxygen and nutrients can pass from the mother's blood into that of the fetus, and waste products can pass in the reverse direction. The placenta is expelled from the uterus at the birth of the fetus, when it is often called the afterbirth. Marsupials and monotremes do not develop placentas.

The placenta: Our least understood organ. Penn Medicine. (n.d.). https://www.pennmedicine.org/news/news-blog/2016/january/the-placenta-our-least-underst

Infarcts - an area of tissue that undergoes necrosis, as a result of obstruction of local blood supply (death of cells of tissue).

The placenta and its health are vital to the health of a woman's pregnancy and fetal development. This organ provides oxygen, nutrients, and filters fetal waste during pregnancy.

Placental infarcts are areas of dead tissue found within the placenta, typically caused by blood vessel complications.

This placental abnormality decreases blood flow to the affected areas. At times, this can cause fetal growth restriction or death. Placental infarcts are more commonly experienced by women with severe high blood pressure.

MediLexicon International. (n.d.). What disorders can affect the placenta during pregnancy?. Medical News Today. https://www.medicalnewstoday.com/articles/309618

Necrosis: What Is Necrosis? Types & Causes - Cleveland Clinic

Necrosis is the death of the cells in your body tissues. Necrosis can occur due to injuries, infections or diseases. Lack of blood flow to your tissues and extreme environmental conditions can also cause necrosis. While dead body tissue can be removed, it can't be brought back to good health.

professional, C. C. medical. (n.d.-b). Necrosis: What is necrosis? types & causes. Cleveland Clinic. https://my.clevelandclinic.org/health/diseases/23959-necrosis

Postpartum Hemorrhage: Causes, Risks, Diagnosis & Treatment

Your placenta attaches to the wall of your uterus and provides food and oxygen to your baby during pregnancy. After your baby is delivered, your uterus continues to contract to deliver the placenta. This is called the third stage of labor. Contractions also help to compress the blood vessels where the placenta was attached to your uterine wall.

professional, C. C. medical. (n.d.-b). Postpartum hemorrhage: Causes, risks, diagnosis & treatment. Cleveland Clinic. https://my.clevelandclinic.org/health/diseases/22228-postpartum-hemorrhage

Amniocentesis (AFT): Sampling of amniotic fluid for genetic conditions including the assessment of infection of and fetal lung maturity.

Alpha-Fetoprotein Test | American Pregnancy Association

The Alpha-Fetoprotein Test (AFT) test is a screening test that examines the level of alpha-fetoprotein in the mother's blood during pregnancy. This is not a diagnostic test. ... If the testing still maintains abnormal results, a more invasive procedure such as amniocentesis may be performed.

Editor. (2022, May 5). Alpha-Fetoprotein Test (AFP). American Pregnancy Association. https://americanpregnancy.org/prenatal-testing/alpha-fetoprotein-test/

Oligohydramnios: Deficiency of amniotic fluid in the amniotic sac. Amniotic fluid is necessary to allow for normal fetal movement, lung development, and cushioning from uterine compression. Low amniotic fluid can be attributed to a maternal, fetal, placental or idiopathic cause resulting in poor fetal outcomes including death.

Wikimedia Foundation. (2022, December 12). Oligohydramnios. Wikipedia. https://en.wikipedia.org/wiki/Oligohydramnios

Idiopathic: Relating to or denoting any disease or condition which arises spontaneously or for which the cause is unknown: idiopathic epilepsy.

Merriam-Webster. (n.d.). Idiopathic definition & meaning. Merriam-Webster. https://www.merriam-webster.com/dictionary/idiopathic

Amniotic fluid: Is the protective liquid contained by the amniotic sac of a gravity amniotic. This fluid, but also serves to facilitate the exchange of nutrients, water, and biochemical products between mother and fetus.

Merriam-Webster. (n.d.). Idiopathic definition & meaning. Merriam-Webster. https://www.merriam-webster.com/dictionary/idiopathic

Deep tendon

Chapter 72Deep Tendon Reflexes

Walker HK.

Publication Details

Definition

In a normal person, when a muscle tendon is tapped briskly, the muscle immediately contracts due to a two-neuron reflex arc involving the spinal or brain stem segment that innervates the muscle. The afferent neuron whose cell body lies in a dorsal root ganglion innervates the muscle or Golgi tendon organ associated with the muscles; the afferent neuron is an alpha motoneuron in the anterior horn of the cord. The cerebral cortex and a number of brainstem nuclei exert influence over the sensory input of the muscle spindles by means of the gamma motoneurons that are located in the anterior horn; these neurons supply a set of muscle fibers that control the length of the muscle spindle itself.

Hyporeflexia is an absent or diminished response to tapping. It usually indicates a disease that involves one or more of the components of the two-neuron reflex arc itself.

Hyperreflexia refers to hyperactive or repeating (clonic) reflexes. These usually indicate an interruption of corticospinal and other descending pathways that influence the reflex arc due to a suprasegmental lesion, that is, a lesion above the level of the spinal reflex pathways.

By convention the deep tendon reflexes are graded as follows:

0 = no response; always abnormal
1+ = a slight but definitely present response; may or may not be normal
2+ = a brisk response; normal
3+ = a very brisk response; may or may not be normal
4+ = a tap elicits a repeating reflex (clonus); always abnormal

Whether the 1 + and 3 + responses are normal depends on what they were previously, that is, the patient's reflex history; what the other reflexes are; and analysis of associated findings such as muscle tone, muscle strength, or other evidence of disease. Asymmetry of reflexes suggests abnormality.

Deep tendon reflexes - clinical methods - NCBI bookshelf. (n.d.). https://www.ncbi.nlm.nih.gov/books/NBK396/

Things to know

Sign

What is hyperreflexia a sign of

Hyperreflexia (brisk reflexes) – reflexes that are faster than normal, jumpy, and seem "trigger happy" – is a common anxiety disorder symptom, including anxiety and panic attacks, generalized anxiety disorder, social anxiety disorder, obsessive-compulsive disorder, phobias, and others.

Anxiety and hyperreflexia. AnxietyCentre.com. (2022, March 12). https://www.anxietycentre.com/anxiety-disorders/symptoms/hyperreflexia/

Original communication

Amnion nodosum:

A lesion of the placenta apparently associated with deficient secretion of fetal urine

Author links open overlay panelBenjamin H. Landing M.D., Boston, Mass. a b
A
Department of Pathology, Boston Lying-in Hospital, USA
B
Harvard Medical School, USA
Available online 25 April 2016, Version of Record 25 April 2016.

Show less
Add to Mendeley
Share
Cite
https://doi.org/10.1016/0002-9378(50)90016-0
Get rights and content

Abstract

Amnion nodosum is a process characterized by multiple, focal lesions of the amnion, consisting of masses of adherent amniotic squamae partially invaded by amniotic mesoderm. The nodules thus formed have previously been called Amnionknötchen (amniotic nodules). This report is based on a study of amnion nodosum occurring in the placentas of eight stillborn infants or infants with major congenital renal anomalies. The study suggests that amnion nodosum is the result of processes set under way by oligohydramnios, caused most commonly by deficiency of fetal urine excretion.

Author links open overlay panelBenjamin H. Landing M.D., a, b, & AbstractAmnion nodosum is a process characterized by multiple. (2016, April 25). Amnion nodosum: A lesion of the placenta apparently associated with deficient secretion of fetal urine. American Journal of Obstetrics and Gynecology. https://www.sciencedirect.com/science/article/pii/0002937850900160

Cited by (13)

Criteria for placental examination for obstetrical and neonatal providers

2023, American Journal of Obstetrics and Gynecology
Show abstract
Experimental production of pulmonary hypoplasia following amniocentesis and oligohydramnios
1983, Early Human Development
Show abstract
Perinatal mortality and morbidity: The role of the anatomical pathologist
1986, Seminars in Perinatology
Early and Late Membrane / Amnion Rupture and Amnion Nodosum
2018, Placental and Gestational Pathology
Pleura nodosum: Fetal squamous debris in an unusual location
2015, Pediatric and Developmental Pathology
Pathology of the human placenta, sixth edition
2012, Pathology of the Human Placenta
View all citing articles on Scopus
View full text
Home U.S. Commission on Civil Rights Since 1957
Racial disparities in maternal health. Racial Disparities in Maternal Health | U.S. Commission on Civil Rights. (n.d.-a). https://www.usccr.gov/reports/2021/racial-disparities-maternal-health

HARVARD HEALTH BLOG

A soaring maternal mortality rate: What does it mean for you?

October 16, 2018

By Neel Shah, MD, MPP, FACOG, Contributor

Neel Shah, M. (2018, October 16). A soaring maternal mortality rate: What does it mean for you?. Harvard Health. https://www.health.harvard.edu/blog/a-soaring-maternal-mortality-rate-what-does-it-mean-for-you-2018101614914

YouTube. (2019). Closing the maternal mortality gap & improving outcomes for mothers. YouTube. Retrieved June 1, 2023, from https://www.youtube.com/watch?v=kMZlfC0297s&t=10s.

LINKS

Centers for Disease Control and Prevention. (2023, February 27). NVSS - Vital Statistics Reporting Guidance. Centers for Disease Control and Prevention. https://www.cdc.gov/nchs/nvss/reporting-guidance.htm

A Reference Guide for Certification of Deaths Associated With Pregnancy on Death Certificates

This reference guide provides physicians, medical examiners, coroners, and other medical certifiers with specific recommendations and examples of documenting different types of deaths associated with pregnancy. Series: Vital Statistics Reporting Guidance; no. 4 Document Type: Report Genre: Statistics Place as Subject: United States Collection(s):

Centers for Disease Control and Prevention. (n.d.-a). A reference guide for certification of deaths associated with pregnancy on death certificates. Centers for Disease Control and Prevention. https://stacks.cdc.gov/view/cdc/114453

Pregnancy-related Deaths | VitalSigns | CDC

Overview Every pregnancy-related death is tragic, especially because about 60% are preventable. Still, about 700 women die each year from complications of pregnancy. A pregnancy-related death can happen during pregnancy, at delivery, and even up to a year afterward (postpartum). For 2011-2015: about 1/3 of deaths (31%) happened during pregnancy;

Centers for Disease Control and Prevention. (n.d.). Number 1 cause of death during Pregnancy. Centers for Disease Control and Prevention. https://www.cdc.gov/vitalsigns/maternal-deaths/index.html

Centers for Disease Control and Prevention. (2023b, March 16). Maternal mortality rates in the United States, 2021. Centers for Disease Control and Prevention. https://www.cdc.gov/nchs/data/hestat/maternal-mortality/2021/maternal-mortality-rates-2021.htm

(DCD), D. C. D. (2023, April 20). How can I complain about poor medical care I received in a hospital?. HHS.gov. https://www.hhs.gov/answers/health-insurance-reform/how-can-i-complain-about-poor-medical-care/index.html

Pregnancy Mortality Surveillance System | Maternal and Infant Health | CDC

The Pregnancy Mortality Surveillance System (PMSS) defines a pregnancy-related death as the death of a woman while pregnant or within 1 year of the end of pregnancy from any cause related to or aggravated by the pregnancy.

https://www.cdc.gov/.../maternal-mortality/pregnancy-mortality-surveillance-system.htm

Centers for Disease Control and Prevention. (2023c, March 23). Pregnancy mortality surveillance system. Centers for Disease Control and Prevention. https://www.cdc.gov/reproductivehealth/maternal-mortality/pregnancy-mortality-surveillance-system.htm

Maternal Mortality - Centers for Disease Control and Prevention

Pregnancy Mortality Surveillance System CDC conducts national surveillance of pregnancy-related deaths to learn more about the causes of pregnancy-related deaths and risk factors associated with these deaths. Prevention Learn more about helping prevent pregnancy-related death, risk factors, what CDC is doing, and other resources.

https://www.cdc.gov/reproductivehealth/maternal-mortality/pregnancy-mortality-surveillance-system.htm

Pregnancy-related Deaths | VitalSigns | CDC

Overview Every pregnancy-related death is tragic, especially because about 60% are preventable. Still, about 700 women die each year from complications of pregnancy. A pregnancy-related death can happen during pregnancy, at delivery, and even up to a year afterward (postpartum). For 2011-2015: about 1/3 of deaths (31%) happened during pregnancy;

Global Health Observatory - World Health Organization (WHO)

In this portal you will find the most up to date global health data, including regional and country data organized separately in the areas of maternal, newborn, child and adolescent health. The data can be visualized on charts and maps which you can download. Global Strategy for Women's, Children's and Adolescents' Health (2016-2030)

World Health Organization. (n.d.). Global health observatory. World Health Organization. https://www.who.int/data/gho

Maternal and reproductive health - World Health Organization (WHO)

295 000 women died of maternal causes in 2017 Antenatal care 75% of pregnant women (in 75 countries with data since 2009) had at least 4 antenatal care visits Family planning 77% of women of reproductive age who are married or in-union have their need for family planning met with a modern method More maternal and reproductive health data products

World Health Organization. (n.d.-b). Maternal and reproductive health. World Health Organization. https://www.who.int/data/gho/data/themes/maternal-and-reproductive-health

Number of maternal deaths - World Health Organization (WHO)

Recorded or estimated number of maternal deaths. Measurement requires information on pregnancy status, timing of death (during pregnancy, childbirth, or within 42 days of termination of pregnancy), and cause of death. Links: Trends in Maternal Mortality: 2000 to 2017 (WHO, UNICEF, UNFPA, World Bank Group and the United Nations Population Division)

World Health Organization. (n.d.-c). Number of maternal deaths. World Health Organization. https://www.who.int/data/gho/data/indicators/indicator-details/GHO/number-of-maternal-deaths

About

Dr. Neel Shah, MD, MPP, FACOG, is Chief Medical Officer of Maven Clinic, the world's largest virtual clinic for family health care. He is also a visiting scientist at Harvard Medical School where he previously served as a professor of obstetrics, gynecology and reproductive biology.

Dr. Shah has been recognized with the Franklin Delano Roosevelt Humanitarian of the Year Award from the March of Dimes for his impact on maternal health in the United States. He is featured in the films Aftershock, which won the Special Jury Prize for Impact at the 2022 Sundance Film Festival, and The Color of Care from the Smithsonian Channel and Executive Producer Oprah Winfrey. Dr. Shah founded the nonprofits Costs of Care and March for Moms, as well as the Delivery Decisions Initiative at Ariadne Labs, a research and social impact program of the Harvard T.H. Chan School of Public Health.

As a physician-scientist, Dr. Shah has written landmark academic papers on maternal health and health care policy, and contributed to four books, including as senior author of Understanding Value-Based Healthcare (McGraw-Hill), which industry leaders have called "an instant classic" and "a masterful primer for all clinicians." He is listed among the "40 smartest people in health care" by the Becker's Hospital Review. Dr. Shah currently serves on the advisory board of the National Institutes of Health, Office of Women's Health Research.

Neel Shah - Chief medical officer - maven clinic | linkedin. (n.d.-b). https://www.linkedin.com/in/neeltshah

National Maternal Mental Health Hotline | MCHB

The National Maternal Mental Health Hotline can help. Call or text 1-833-943-5746 (1-833-9-HELP4MOMS). TTY users can use a preferred relay service or dial 711 and then 1-833-943-5746. If you are in suicidal crisis, please call or text 988 or visit the 988 Suicide & Crisis Lifeline. Pregnancy and a new baby can bring a range of emotions.

National Maternal Mental Health hotline. MCHB. (n.d.). https://mchb.hrsa.gov/national-maternal-mental-health-hotline

Postpartum Support International - PSI

1-800-944-4773 #1 En Español or #2 English Text "Help" to 800-944-4773 (EN) Text en Español: 971-203-7773 Get Help 988 Suicide & Crisis Lifeline National Maternal Mental Health Hotline (US only) *The PSI HelpLine does not handle emergencies. People in crisis should call their local emergency number or the Suicide & Crisis Lifeline at 988.

Postpartum support international - psi. Postpartum Support International (PSI). (2023, April 26). https://www.postpartum.net/

Postpartum Recovery - American Pregnancy Association

Postpartum Recovery. The first six weeks after the delivery of your baby are considered your "recovery" period, eight weeks if you had a cesarean section. But some believe recovery lasts for six months up to one year postpartum. Even if you had the easiest delivery on record (and especially if you didn't), your body has been stretched and stressed, so it needs time to recover and regroup.

Editor. (2021, December 9). Postpartum recovery. American Pregnancy Association. https://americanpregnancy.org/healthy-pregnancy/first-year-of-life/postpartum-recovery/

2023 Black Maternal Health Week - Black Mamas Matter Alliance

Held annually on April 11-17th, BMHW is a week-long campaign founded and led by the Black Mamas Matter Alliance to build awareness, activism, and community-building to amplify the voices, perspectives and lived experiences of Black Mamas and birthing people.

2023 Black Maternal Health Week. Black Mamas Matter Alliance. (2023, April 7). https://blackmamasmatter.org/2023-black-maternal-health-week/

Black Maternal Health Week - California Department of Public Health

Black Maternal Health Week Home Programs Center for Family Health Maternal, Child and Adolescent Health Division Black Maternal Health Week Maternal, CHild and Adolescent Health Division Forbidden Black Maternal Health Week April 11–17 Copy and paste the text to share on Facebook, Twitter or Instagram.

https://www.cdph.ca.gov/.../DMCAH/Pages/Health-Observances/Black-Maternal-Health-Week.aspx

#BMHW21: CAMPAIGN TOOLKIT - Black Mamas Matter Alliance

Monday April 12, 2021 3:30pm – 4:30pm EST Sample Facebook & Instagram Posts It's important to elevate Black Mamas' voices and perspectives around issues that impact them. Black Mamas are best situated to solve the challenges in their communities.

#BMHW21: Campaign toolkit. Black Mamas Matter Alliance. (2022, April 13). https://blackmamasmatter.org/bmhw22/toolkit/

Secretary Becerra and HHS Leaders Celebrate Black Maternal Health Week ...

Biden-Harris Administration continues to advance its goals of improving maternal health and equity. Today, Secretary Xavier Becerra and leaders across the U.S. Department of Health and Human Services (HHS) released the following statements in recognition of Black Maternal Health Week, which takes place this year from April 11 –17.

Assistant Secretary for Public Affairs (ASPA). (2023, January 20). Secretary Becerra and HHS leaders celebrate Black Maternal Health Week 2022. HHS.gov. https://www.hhs.gov/about/news/2022/04/11/secretary-becerra-and-hhs-leaders-celebrate-black-maternal-health-week-2022.html

What Is A Midwife, And What Do They Do? – Forbes Health

Like a physician, a midwife attends labor and delivery to safely bring a new baby into the world. In low-risk pregnancies, a midwife can autonomously deliver in a hospital, birthing center or a family's home.

Forbes Magazine. (2023, April 28). What is a midwife?. Forbes. https://www.forbes.com/health/family/what-is-a-midwife/

What is a doula and what do they do? - Medical News Today

The role of a doula. The doula's role is to provide practical and emotional support to a pregnant individual, their partner, and family members. During a person's pregnancy, a doula will spend time building a trusting relationship with them. They will support them, help them create a birth plan, and answer their questions.

MediLexicon International. (n.d.-d). What is a Doula and what do they do?. Medical News Today. https://www.medicalnewstoday.com/articles/what-is-a-doula

Trauma in Pregnancy: Assessment, Management, and Prevention

Trauma complicates one in 12 pregnancies, and is the leading non-obstetric cause of death among pregnant women. 1 – 3 Traumatic injuries to pregnant women are unintentional motor vehicle crashes, assaults, falls, and intimate partner violence.

Murphy, N. J., & Quinlan, J. D. (2014, November 15). Trauma in pregnancy: Assessment, management, and prevention. American Family Physician. https://www.aafp.org/pubs/afp/issues/2014/1115/p717.html

Patient Safety: What You Can Do to Be a Safe Patient

5 Tips for Patients [Video – 2:32] Protect yourself and your family from harmful germs that can cause infections Keep your hands clean. Regular hand cleaning is one of the best ways to remove germs, avoid getting sick, and prevent spreading germs. Take antibiotics only when your provider thinks you need them. Ask if your antibiotic is necessary.

Centers for Disease Control and Prevention. (2019, November 6). Patient safety: What you can do to be a safe patient. Centers for Disease Control and Prevention. https://www.cdc.gov/hai/patientsafety/patient-safety.html

Everything You Need To Know About The Freedom Of Information Law

The New York State Freedom of Information Law, outlined in Article 6 of the New York Public Officers Law, was enacted in 1974 to make government more transparent for New Yorkers.

David CruzPublished Sep 11, 2021ShareFacebookTwitterRedditEmail, & James RamsayPublished Jun 2, 2023 at 2:09 p.m. (n.d.). Everything you need to know about the freedom of information law. Gothamist. https://gothamist.com/news/everything-you-need-know-freedom-of-information-law-foil-explainer

The Freedom of Information Act, 5 U.S.C. § 552

§ 552. Public information; agency rules, opinions, orders, records, and proceedings. Each agency shall make available to the public   information as follows: (1) Each agency shall separately state and currently publish in the Federal Register for the guidance of the   public—The Freedom of Information Act, 5 U.S.C. § 552. The United States Department of Justice. (2022, January 21). https://www.justice.gov/oip/freedom-information-act-5-usc-552

`20/20' Transcript Reveals Patients' Stories Of Pain The Following Is A ...

`20/20' Transcript Reveals Patients' Stories Of Pain The Following Is A Transcript Of The Sept. 11 "20/20" Show About Former Hazleton-st. Joseph Medical Center Dr. Frank Ruhl Peterson,...

Times Leader Archivist, By, & Archivist, T. L. (2021, February 20). `20/20' transcript reveals patients' stories of pain the following is a transcript of the Sept. 11 "20/20" show about former Hazleton-St. Joseph Medical Center dr. Frank Ruhl Peterson, who pleaded guilty to charges that he took drugs intended for patients while he worked at the hospital and Conyngham Anesthesia Associates. Times Leader. https://www.timesleader.com/archive/919549/20-20-transcript-reveals-patients-stories-of-pain-the-following-is-a-transcript-of-the-sept-11-20-20-show-about-former-hazleton-st-joseph-medical-center-dr-frank-ruhl-peterson-who-ple

Some Health Workers Suffering From Addiction Steal Drugs Meant For Patients

Listen · 4:59 4-Minute Listen Playlist Download Embed Transcript Enlarge this image The federal government estimates one in 10 healthcare workers experience substance use disorder. There is...

Mann, B. (2020, October 5). Some health workers suffering from addiction steal drugs meant for patients. NPR.   https://www.npr.org/2020/10/05/918279481/some-health-workers-suffering-from-addiction-steal-drugs-meant-for-patients

Addiction and Substance Abuse in Anesthesiology

A review of 1,000 treated physicians conducted by Talbott et al .9in 1987 suggested that addiction is common among anesthesiologists. Anesthesia residents represented 33.7% of all residents presenting for treatment but composed only 4.6% of all US resident physicians at the time of the study, thus presenting an apparent 7.4-fold increased prevalence of anesthesia residents in the study …

Bryson, E., Silverstein, J., Warner, D., & Warner, M. (2008, November 1). Addiction and substance abuse in anesthesiology. American Society of Anesthesiologists. https://pubs.asahq.org/anesthesiology/article/109/5/905/9097/Addiction-and-Substance-Abuse-in-Anesthesiology

HARVARD HEALTH BLOG

A soaring maternal mortality rate: What does it mean for you?

October 16, 2018

By Neel Shah, MD, MPP, FACOG, Contributor

Neel Shah, M. (2018, October 16). A soaring maternal mortality rate: What does it mean for you?. Harvard Health. https://www.health.harvard.edu/blog/a-soaring-maternal-mortality-rate-what-does-it-mean-for-you-2018101614914

YouTube. (2019). Closing the maternal mortality gap & improving outcomes for mothers. YouTube. Retrieved June 1, 2023, from https://www.youtube.com/watch?v=kMZlfC0297s&t=10s.

REFERENCES

#BMHW21: Campaign toolkit. Black Mamas Matter Alliance. (2022a, April 13). https://blackmamasmatter. org/bmhw22/toolkit/

#BMHW21: Campaign toolkit. Black Mamas Matter Alliance. (2022b, April 13). https://blackmamasmatter. org/bmhw22/toolkit/

(DCD), D. C. D. (2023, April 20). *How can I complain about poor medical care I received in a hospital?.* HHS.gov. https://www.hhs.gov/answers/health-insurance-reform/how-can-i-complain-about-poor-medical-care/index.html

2023 Black Maternal Health Week. Black Mamas Matter Alliance. (2023, April 7). https://blackmamasmatter. org/2023-black-maternal-health-week/

Aggeler, M. (2018, August 6). *Beyoncé opens up about her difficult pregnancy and emergency C-section.* The Cut. https://www.thecut.com/2018/08/beyonce-vogue-september-issue-twins-childbirth-c-section. html

AM;, A. C. (n.d.). *Ischemic placental disease and risks of perinatal mortality and morbidity and neurodevelopmental outcomes.* Seminars in perinatology. https://pubmed.ncbi.nlm.nih.gov/24836827/

Anxiety and hyperreflexia. AnxietyCentre.com. (2022, March 12). https://www.anxietycentre.com/ anxiety-disorders/symptoms/hyperreflexia/

Assistant Secretary for Public Affairs (ASPA). (2023, January 20). *Secretary Becerra and HHS leaders celebrate Black Maternal Health Week 2022.* HHS.gov. https://www.hhs.gov/about/news/2022/04/11/ secretary-becerra-and-hhs-leaders-celebrate-black-maternal-health-week-2022.html

Author links open overlay panelBenjamin H. Landing M.D., a, b, & AbstractAmnion nodosum is a process characterized by multiple. (2016, April 25). *Amnion nodosum: A lesion of the placenta apparently associated with deficient secretion of fetal urine.* American Journal of Obstetrics and Gynecology. https:// www.sciencedirect.com/science/article/pii/0002937850900160

Author links open overlay panelMariele Gatto, AbstractPrimary systemic vasculitis are uncommon diseases that may affect young women in their childbearing age. To date, Ishikawa, K., Wong, V. C. W., Sharma, B. K., Grewal, K., Rocha, M. P., Hampl, J. C., Herrema, I., Winn, H. N., Chua, S., Askie, L. M., Sibai, B., Nagey, D. A., Owen, J., Aya, A. G., Dayoan, E. S., Bessias, N., M'Rad, S., ... Graca, L.

M. (2011, December 3). *Pregnancy and vasculitis: A systematic review of the literature.* Autoimmunity Reviews. https://www.sciencedirect.com/science/article/abs/pii/S156899721100293X

Betamethasone injection uses, side effects & warnings. Drugs.com. (n.d.-a). https://www.drugs.com/mtm/betamethasone-injection.html

Centers for Disease Control and Prevention. (2019, November 6). *Patient safety: What you can do to be a safe patient.* Centers for Disease Control and Prevention. https://www.cdc.gov/hai/patientsafety/patient-safety.html

Centers for Disease Control and Prevention. (2020a, May 4). *Patient safety.* Centers for Disease Control and Prevention. https://www.cdc.gov/patientsafety/index.html

Centers for Disease Control and Prevention. (2020b, May 4). *Patient safety.* Centers for Disease Control and Prevention. https://www.cdc.gov/patientsafety/index.html

Centers for Disease Control and Prevention. (2020c, July 27). *Rheumatoid arthritis (RA).* Centers for Disease Control and Prevention. https://www.cdc.gov/arthritis/basics/rheumatoid-arthritis.html

Centers for Disease Control and Prevention. (2022, July 5). *Systemic lupus erythematosus (SLE).* Centers for Disease Control and Prevention. https://www.cdc.gov/lupus/facts/detailed.html

Centers for Disease Control and Prevention. (2023a, February 27). *NVSS - Vital Statistics Reporting Guidance.* Centers for Disease Control and Prevention. https://www.cdc.gov/nchs/nvss/reporting-guidance.htm

Centers for Disease Control and Prevention. (2023b, March 16). *Maternal mortality rates in the United States, 2021.* Centers for Disease Control and Prevention. https://www.cdc.gov/nchs/data/hestat/maternal-mortality/2021/maternal-mortality-rates-2021.htm

Centers for Disease Control and Prevention. (2023c, March 23). *Pregnancy mortality surveillance system.* Centers for Disease Control and Prevention. https://www.cdc.gov/reproductivehealth/maternal-mortality/pregnancy-mortality-surveillance-system.htm

Centers for Disease Control and Prevention. (2023d, March 23). *Pregnancy mortality surveillance system.* Centers for Disease Control and Prevention. https://www.cdc.gov/reproductivehealth/maternal-mortality/pregnancy-mortality-surveillance-system.htm

Centers for Disease Control and Prevention. (2023e, March 23). *Pregnancy mortality surveillance system.* Centers for Disease Control and Prevention. https://www.cdc.gov/reproductivehealth/maternal-mortality/pregnancy-mortality-surveillance-system.htm

Centers for Disease Control and Prevention. (n.d.-a). *A reference guide for certification of deaths associated with pregnancy on death certificates.* Centers for Disease Control and Prevention. https://stacks.cdc.gov/view/cdc/114453

Centers for Disease Control and Prevention. (n.d.-b). *Number 1 cause of death during Pregnancy.* Centers for Disease Control and Prevention. https://www.cdc.gov/vitalsigns/maternal-deaths/index.html

Cheryl Bird, R. (2021, June 14). *Magnesium sulfate and premature labor.* Verywell Family. https://www.verywellfamily.com/magnesium-sulfate-in-preterm-labor-2748458

Cirino, E. (2018, September 12). *Treatment of preeclampsia: Magnesium sulfate therapy.* Healthline. https://www.healthline.com/health/pregnancy/preeclampsia-magnesium-sulfate-therapy

David CruzPublished Sep 11, 2021ShareFacebookTwitterRedditEmail, & James RamsayPublished Jun 2, 2023 at 2:09 p.m. (n.d.). *Everything you need to know about the freedom of information law.* Gothamist. https://gothamist.com/news/everything-you-need-know-freedom-of-information-law-foil-explainer

Deep tendon reflexes - clinical methods - NCBI bookshelf. (n.d.-a). https://www.ncbi.nlm.nih.gov/books/NBK396/

Editor. (2021, December 9). *Postpartum recovery.* American Pregnancy Association. https://americanpregnancy.org/healthy-pregnancy/first-year-of-life/postpartum-recovery/

Editor. (2022, May 5). *Alpha-Fetoprotein Test (AFP).* American Pregnancy Association. https://americanpregnancy.org/prenatal-testing/alpha-fetoprotein-test/

Editors, H. (2022, June 22). *It's not normal: Black women, stop suffering from fibroids.* HealthyWomen. https://www.healthywomen.org/content/article/its-not-normal-black-women-stop-suffering-fibroids

Fibroids: The 411. CARE About Fibroids. (n.d.). http://www.careaboutfibroids.org/411.html

Forbes Magazine. (2023, April 28). *What is a midwife?.* Forbes. https://www.forbes.com/health/family/what-is-a-midwife/

The Freedom of Information Act, 5 U.S.C. § 552. The United States Department of Justice. (2022, January 21). https://www.justice.gov/oip/freedom-information-act-5-usc-552

Gangstarrgirl. (2020, March 28). *Bakari Sellers' wife Ellen almost lost her life while giving birth to twins.* MadameNoire. https://madamenoire.com/1062109/bakari-sellers-wife-ellen-almost-lost-her-life-while-giving-birth-to-twins/

Gatto M;Iaccarino L;Canova M;Zen M;Nalotto L;Ramonda R;Punzi L;Doria A; (n.d.). *Pregnancy and vasculitis: A systematic review of the literature.* Autoimmunity reviews. https://pubmed.ncbi.nlm.nih.gov/22155197/

Health, D. of P. (n.d.). Black Maternal Health Week. https://www.cdph.ca.gov/Programs/CFH/DMCAH/Pages/Health-Observances/Black-Maternal-Health-Week.aspx

Institute of Medicine of Chicago - new report: Racial disparities in maternal health U.S. Commission on Civil Rights 2021 Statutory Enforcement Report. (n.d.). https://iomc.org/news/11097557

Macon, B. L. (2018, September 12). *Eclampsia: Causes, symptoms, and diagnosis.* Healthline. https://www.healthline.com/health/eclampsia

Magnesium sulfate use during pregnancy. Drugs.com. (n.d.-b). https://www.drugs.com/pregnancy/magnesium-sulfate.html

Marcoux, H. (2021, December 16). *Olympian Allyson Felix recalls the scariest day of her life. it was the day she gave birth.* Insider. https://www.insider.com/allyson-felix-opened-up-about-her-traumatic-birth-2021-12

Mauch, A. (2020, July 10). *Death of pregnant black woman, sha-asia washington, highlights racial disparities in maternal mortality.* Peoplemag. https://people.com/health/death-of-pregnant-black-woman-sha-asia-washington-highlights-racial-disparities-in-maternal-mortality/

Mayo Foundation for Medical Education and Research. (2021, August 17). *Postpartum preeclampsia.* Mayo Clinic. https://www.mayoclinic.org/diseases-conditions/postpartum-preeclampsia/diagnosis-treatment/drc-20376652

Mayo Foundation for Medical Education and Research. (2022a, April 15). *Gestational proteinuria Preeclampsia review.* Mayo Clinic. https://www.mayoclinic.org/diseases-conditions/preeclampsia/symptoms-causes/syc-20355745

Mayo Foundation for Medical Education and Research. (2022b, April 15). *Preeclampsia.* Mayo Clinic. https://www.mayoclinic.org/diseases-conditions/preeclampsia/symptoms-causes/syc-20355745

Mayo Foundation for Medical Education and Research. (2022c, April 15). *Preeclampsia.* Mayo Clinic. https://www.mayoclinic.org/diseases-conditions/preeclampsia/symptoms-causes/syc-20355745

Mayo Foundation for Medical Education and Research. (2023, February 16). *General anesthesia.* Mayo Clinic. https://www.mayoclinic.org/tests-procedures/anesthesia/about/pac-20384568

MediLexicon International. (n.d.-a). *Thrombosis: Types, symptoms, treatment, and more.* Medical News Today. https://www.medicalnewstoday.com/articles/thrombosis

MediLexicon International. (n.d.-b). *Thrombosis vs. embolism: Differences, symptoms, and more.* Medical News Today. https://www.medicalnewstoday.com/articles/thrombosis-vs-embolism

MediLexicon International. (n.d.-c). *What disorders can affect the placenta during pregnancy?.* Medical News Today. https://www.medicalnewstoday.com/articles/309618

MediLexicon International. (n.d.-d). *What is a Doula and what do they do?.* Medical News Today. https://www.medicalnewstoday.com/articles/what-is-a-doula

Merriam-Webster. (n.d.-a). *Idiopathic definition & meaning.* Merriam-Webster. https://www.merriam-webster.com/dictionary/idiopathic

Merriam-Webster. (n.d.-b). *Morbidity definition & meaning.* Merriam-Webster. https://www.merriam-webster.com/dictionary/morbidity

Murphy, N. J., & Quinlan, J. D. (2014a, November 15). *Trauma in pregnancy: Assessment, management, and prevention.* American Family Physician. https://www.aafp.org/pubs/afp/issues/2014/1115/p717.html

Murphy, N. J., & Quinlan, J. D. (2014b, November 15). *Trauma in pregnancy: Assessment, management, and prevention.* American Family Physician. https://www.aafp.org/pubs/afp/issues/2014/1115/p717.html

National Maternal Mental Health hotline. MCHB. (n.d.). https://mchb.hrsa.gov/national-maternal-mental-health-hotline

Neel Shah - Chief medical officer - maven clinic | linkedin. (n.d.-b). https://www.linkedin.com/in/neeltshah

Neel Shah, M. (2018, October 16). *A soaring maternal mortality rate: What does it mean for you?*. Harvard Health. https://www.health.harvard.edu/blog/a-soaring-maternal-mortality-rate-what-does-it-mean-for-you-2018101614914

Patient non-compliance- a powerful legal defense. Self-Insurance Programs. (2015, March 13). https://flbog.sip.ufl.edu/risk-rx-article/patient-non-compliance-a-powerful-legal-defense/

Physiology, deep tendon reflexes - statpearls - NCBI bookshelf. (n.d.-c). https://www.ncbi.nlm.nih.gov/books/NBK562238/

The placenta: Our least understood organ. Penn Medicine. (n.d.). https://www.pennmedicine.org/news/news-blog/2016/january/the-placenta-our-least-underst

Poole, S. M. (2018, March 9). *TV judge Glenda Hatchett and Son Fight for lives of New Mothers*. ajc. https://www.ajc.com/marketing/judge-glenda-hatchett-and-son-raise-awareness-maternal-deaths/Z5Jg8DcqSz4NQLMKpP6PML/

Postpartum support international - psi. Postpartum Support International (PSI). (2023, April 26). https://www.postpartum.net/

Products. Cook Medical. (2021a, May 13). https://www.cookmedical.com/products/wh_dan_webds/

Products. Cook Medical. (2021b, May 13). https://www.cookmedical.com/products/wh_dan_webds/

professional, C. C. medical. (n.d.-a). *Amniocentesis: Purpose, procedure, risks, Recovery & Results*. Cleveland Clinic. https://my.clevelandclinic.org/health/treatments/4206-genetic-amniocentesis

professional, C. C. medical. (n.d.-b). *Eclampsia: Causes, symptoms, diagnosis & treatment*. Cleveland Clinic. https://my.clevelandclinic.org/health/diseases/24333-eclampsia

professional, C. C. medical. (n.d.-c). *Necrosis: What is necrosis? types & causes*. Cleveland Clinic. https://my.clevelandclinic.org/health/diseases/23959-necrosis

professional, C. C. medical. (n.d.-d). *Postpartum hemorrhage: Causes, risks, diagnosis & treatment*. Cleveland Clinic. https://my.clevelandclinic.org/health/diseases/22228-postpartum-hemorrhage

professional, C. C. medical. (n.d.-e). *Thrombosis: What you need to know*. Cleveland Clinic. https://my.clevelandclinic.org/health/diseases/22242-thrombosis

Racial disparities in maternal health. Racial Disparities in Maternal Health | U.S. Commission on Civil Rights. (n.d.-a). https://www.usccr.gov/reports/2021/racial-disparities-maternal-health

Racial disparities in maternal health. Racial Disparities in Maternal Health | U.S. Commission on Civil Rights. (n.d.-b). https://www.usccr.gov/reports/2021/racial-disparities-maternal-health

Rights, U. S. C. on C. (2021, September 15). *U.S. Commission on Civil Rights Releases Report: Racial Disparities in maternal health*. PR Newswire: press release distribution, targeting, monitoring and marketing. https://www.prnewswire.com/news-releases/us-commission-on-civil-rights-releases-report-racial-disparities-in-maternal-health-301377760.html

Rucker Sellers, E. (2019, February 11). *Ellen RUCKER sellers*. Ellen Rucker sellers. http://ellenruckersellers.com/

Seladi-Schulman, J. (2020, November 11). *Morbidity vs. mortality rate: What's the difference?* Healthline. https://www.healthline.com/health/morbidity-vs-mortality

SEVERE PRE ECLAMPSIA . The Joint Commission. (n.d.). https://www.jointcommission.org/resources/patient-safety/

Shomon, M. (n.d.). *Know the symptoms of some common autoimmune conditions*. Verywell Health. https://www.verywellhealth.com/autoimmune-disease-symptoms-3232847

Steroid shots help speed up the development of your baby's lungs, & Miles, K. (n.d.-a). *Betamethasone in pregnancy: How steroid shots can help your baby's lungs*. BabyCenter. https://www.babycenter.com/pregnancy/your-body/should-i-take-steroids-during-preterm-labor_5437

Steroid shots help speed up the development of your baby's lungs, & Miles, K. (n.d.-b). *Betamethasone in pregnancy: How steroid shots can help your baby's lungs*. BabyCenter. https://www.babycenter.com/pregnancy/your-body/should-i-take-steroids-during-preterm-labor_5437

Steroid shots help speed up the development of your baby's lungs, & Miles, K. (n.d.-c). *Betamethasone in pregnancy: How steroid shots can help your baby's lungs*. BabyCenter. https://www.babycenter.com/pregnancy/your-body/should-i-take-steroids-during-preterm-labor_5437

U.S. Commission on Civil Rights Releases Report: Racial Dispariti es in maternal health. U.S. Commission on Civil Rights Releases Report: Racial Disparities in Maternal Health | U.S. Commission on Civil Rights. (n.d.). https://www.usccr.gov/news/2021/us-commi ssion-civil-rights-releases-report-racial-disparities-maternal-health

U.S. National Library of Medicine. (n.d.). *Autoimmune disorders: Medlineplus medical encyclopedia*. MedlinePlus. https://medlineplus.gov/ency/article/000816.htm

The United States Government. (2023, April 10). *A proclamation on Black Maternal Health Week, 2023*. The White House. https://www.whitehouse.gov/briefing-room/presidential-actions/2023/04/10/a-proclamation-on-black-maternal-health-week-2023/

Wikimedia Foundation. (2022, December 12). *Oligohydramnios*. Wikipedia. https://en.wikipedia.org/wiki/Oligohydramnios

Wikimedia Foundation. (2023, April 25). *Amniotic fluid*. Wikipedia. https://en.wikipedia.org/wiki/Amniotic_fluid

Williams, S. (2018, February 20). *Serena Williams: What my life-threatening experience taught me about giving birth*. CNN. https://www.cnn.com/2018/02/20/opinions/protect-mother-pregnancy-williams-opinion/index.html

World Health Organization. (n.d.-a). *Global health observatory*. World Health Organization. https://www.who.int/data/gho

World Health Organization. (n.d.-b). *Maternal and reproductive health*. World Health Organization. https://www.who.int/data/gho/data/themes/maternal-and-reproductive-health

World Health Organization. (n.d.-c). *Number of maternal deaths*. World Health Organization. https://www.who.int/data/gho/data/indicators/indicator-details/GHO/number-of-maternal-deaths

YouTube. (2019). *Closing the maternal mortality gap & improving outcomes for mothers*. YouTube. Retrieved June 1, 2023, from https://www.youtube.com/watch?v=kMZlfC0297s&t=10s.

GLOSSARY A - Z

Anesthetic: a substance that <u>induces</u> <u>insensitivity</u> to pain.

Anesthesia or anaesthesia: is a state of controlled, temporary loss of sensation or awareness that is induced for medical or veterinary purposes.

Autoimmune: is disease in which the body's immune system attacks healthy cells.

Betamethasone: is a steroid that can treat inflammation and many other medical problems.

Bladder Retractor: The Bladder Retractors are urological surgical instruments used for exposing surgical sites by retracting bladder tissue, skin, and muscles.

Blood Crossmatch: Crossmatching is a way for your healthcare provider to test your blood against a donor's to make sure they are fully compatible.

Catheter: a flexible tube <u>inserted</u> <u>through</u> a narrow opening into a body <u>cavity</u>, particularly the <u>bladder</u>.

Caffeine: Caffeine oral solution is used to treat short-term apnea of prematurity when premature babies (infants between 28 and 32 weeks gestational age) stop breathing.

Cesarean Scar: is the scar left over after a surgical delivery

C-section: is another name for a Cesarean delivery.

Complications: High Blood Pressure, also called hypertension, occurs when arteries carrying blood from the heart to the body organs are narrowed.

Confirmed Pregnancy Due Dates: typically the best way to estimate your due date is to count 40 weeks, or 280 days, from the first day of your last menstrual period (LMP).

Contractions: Tightening of uterine muscle fibers that occurs briefly and intermittently throughout pregnancy and more regularly and forcefully during active labor.

Cornual Angle Fibroid: is found in the upper corner of the uterus (corneal region) can occasionally obstruct fallopian tubes and can be a cause of tubal factor subfertility. Similarly, very large fibroids and an enlarged uterine cavity are a cause of not getting pregnant.

Demerol: is used to treat moderate to severe pain (opioid).

Dorsal Supine Position: this position consumes a patient to lie flat on their back, face and abdomen facing upward.

Eclampsia: is severe hypertension.

Edema: Edna means swelling caused by fluid in your body's tissues.

Fibroid Degeneration: is when a Fibroid stops receiving enough nutrients from its blood supply

Foley Catheter: in urology, a Foley is a catheter is a flexible tube that a clinician passes the urethra and bladder to drain urine.

Hemorrhage: an escape blood from a <u>ruptured</u> blood vessel, especially when <u>profuse</u>.

Hip Flexors: The hip flexors are a group of muscles toward the front of the hip.

Hyper-Reflexes: Hyper-reflexia happens when your muscles have increased or overactive reflex response.

Hypertension: A condition in which the force of the blood against the artery walls is too high.

Intra-Operative Care Plan & Potential For Anxiety

Intra-uterine Pregnancy: is a medical condition in which a fertilized sac is implanted in the uterus

Jagged Bikini Scar: a cesarean scar not symmetrically upturned on both ends

Kocher Clamps: a strong forceps for controlling bleeding in surgery having serrated blades with interlocking teeth at the tips.

Magnesium Sulfate: is used in pregnancy to prevent seizures due to worsening pre-eclampsia, to slow or stop preterm labor, and to prevent injuries to a preterm baby's brain.

Mayo Scissors: are used as utility scissors to cut suture, steri-strips, or electrodes.

Metzenbaum Scissors: are surgical scissors designed for cutting delicate tissue and blunt dissection.

Morality: principles concerning the distinction between right and wrong or good and bad behavior.

Morbidity: the condition of suffering from a disease or medical condition.

Mortality: the state of being subject to death.

Operative Report: At its core, an operative report is simply the summary of a surgical procedure that becomes part of the patient's medical record.

Pathology: is the study of the causes and effects of disease or injury.

Placenta: 1 a flattened circular organ in the uterus of pregnant eutherian mammals, nourishing and maintaining the fetus through the umbilical cord.

Planned Pregnancy: Deciding to pursue a pregnancy before the pregnancy.

Pillow: A quality pregnancy pillow can improve the alignment of your spine, back, and hips; relieve pressure while you sleep; and help you wake up with less pain in the morning.

Postoperative: during, related to, or denoting the period following a surgical operation.

Postoperative Diagnosis: the condition of a patient in the period following a surgical operation.

Postpartum Hemorrhage: Excessive bleeding after childbirth.

Causes of postpartum bleeding include loss of tone in the uterine muscles, a bleeding disorder, or the placenta failing to come out completely or tearing.

Pregnancy Operation: A caesarean section (C-section or caesarean) is an operation to deliver a baby through a cut in the abdomen (tummy) and uterus (womb).

Prenatal Visits: Prenatal care is medical care you get during pregnancy.

Pre-eclampsia: a condition in pregnancy characterized by high blood pressure, sometimes with fluid retention and proteinuria.

Preoperative Diagnosis: The Preoperative Diagnosis Section records the surgical diagnosis assigned to the patient before the surgical procedure which is the reason for surgery.

Procedure: Procedures and surgery are two types of medical interventions used to diagnose, treat, or evaluate a condition or illness.

PTSD: Post-traumatic stress disorder is a mental and behavioral disorder that can develop because of exposure to a traumatic event.

Recovery Room: Patients having surgery will be transferred from the operating room to the PACU for their initial recovery from anesthesia.

Scalpel: a knife with a small, sharp, sometimes detachable blade, as used by a surgeon.

Sedation: the administering of a sedative drug to produce a state of calm or sleep.

Sedative: promoting calm or inducing sleep.

Severe Pre-eclampsia: new onset of hypertension typically around the 20 of each week of pregnancy

Shock Hemorrhage: is a condition of reduced tissue perfusion, resulting in the inadequate delivery of oxygen and nutrients that are necessary for cellular function.

Sonography: the analysis of sound using an instrument which produces a <u>graphical</u> representation of its component <u>frequencies</u>.

Supine Position: this position consumes a patient to lie flat on their back, face and abdomen facing upward.

TENS: A transcutaneous electrical nerve stimulator (TENS) sends electrical pulses through the skin to start your body's own painkillers. The electrical pulses can release endorphins and other substances to stop pain signals in the brain. TENS can reduce pain.

Toxemia: occurs after 20 weeks of pregnancy, resulting from high blood pressure and causes high protein levels in the urine and may affect other organs. It can be dangerous to the mother and the developing fetus.

Toradol: is short term to reduce pain in adults. Typically used before or after a medically procedures and after surgery (NSAID).

Treatment: Magnesium Sulfate Therapy.

Tubal Ligation: is a medical sterilization procedure for women who are sure they don't want a future pregnancy.

Urinary Catheter: A urinary catheter is a hollow, partially flexible tube that collects urine from the bladder and leads to a drainage bag. Urinary catheters come in many sizes and types.

Uterine Atony: Uterine atony refers to the inadequate contraction of the corpus uteri myometrial cells in response to endogenous oxytocin release. Postpartum hemorrhage can occur because spiral arteries are uniquely devoid of musculature and dependent on uterine contractions to mechanically squeeze them into hemostasis.

Uterine Incision: is a surgical procedure in which there is an incision made in the mothers abdomen and uterus.

Vesicouterine Peritoneum: is a fold of the peritoneum over the uterus and the bladder, forming a pelvic recess.

STORY LINKS

I became a very stoic personality type regarding this situation and so I closed off and to the point that I didn't follow, nor was I aware that such an implicit bias and pattern of not listening to Black American Woman was happening to others as well. It was the noise of Singer, *Beyonce*, Tennis Star, *Serena Williams*; TV News Analysis, *Bakari Sellers* and wife *Ellen Rucker Seller*; *Judge Hatchett's son,* Charles Johnson and *daughter in law*, Kyira Johnson, including *Sha-Asia Washington* and Olympic Medalist *Allison* Felix— I'm like, what the hell! Plus, many, many others all suffering a traumatic maternal pregnancy, morbidity or mortality issues/problems of some sort.

RELATED STORY LINKS

ELLEN RUCKER SELLERS

I tell my story not for pity but to educate and bring awareness to the voiceless. Black mothers in the US die at 3 to 4 times the rate of white mothers. The disparity between Black maternal mortality rate and white women is appalling. Bakari and I knew the statistics. By God's grace, mercy, and favor, I am able to share my story.

ellenruckersellers.com

URL http://ellenruckersellers.com/ Website title ELLEN RUCKER SELLERS Date accessed May 28, 2023 Date published February 11, 2019

Rucker Sellers, E. (2019, February 11). Ellen RUCKER sellers. Ellen Rucker sellers. http://ellenruckersellers.com/

Bakari Sellers' Wife Ellen Almost Died While Giving Birth To Twins

Earlier this year, North Carolina native Ellen Rucker Sellers gave birth to twins. Her pregnancy, which was high risk, went well, but her labor and delivery had some unexpected complications. What ...

https://madamenoire.com/1062109/bakari-sellers-wife-ellen-almost-lost-her-life-while…

Article title

Bakari Sellers' Wife Ellen Almost Lost Her Life While Giving Birth To Twins URL https://madamenoire.com/1062109/bakari-sellers-wife-ellen-almost-lost-her-life-while-giving-birth-to-twins/ Website title MadameNoire Date accessed May 28, 2023 Date published March 28, 2020

Gangstarrgirl. (2020, March 28). Bakari Sellers' wife Ellen almost lost her life while giving birth to twins. MadameNoire. https://madamenoire.com/1062109/bakari-sellers-wife-ellen-almost-lost-her-life-while-giving-birth-to-twins/

Rucker Sellers, E. (2019, February 11). Ellen RUCKER sellers. Ellen Rucker sellers. http://ellenruckersellers.com/

———————

Article title

Serena Williams Says Her 'Life or Death' Childbirth Experience Required 4 Surgeries

URL

https://www.self.com/story/serena-williams-childbirth-experience Website title SELF Date accessed May 28, 2023 Date published April 07, 2022

Article title

Serena Williams Says Her 'Life or Death' Childbirth Experience Required 4 Surgeries. (Coady)

_____

Article title

Serena Williams: What my life-threatening experience taught me about giving birth

URL

https://www.cnn.com/2018/02/20/opinions/protect-mother-pregnancy-williams-opinion/index.html

Website title CNN

Date accessed

May 28, 2023

Date published

February 20, 2018

Online publication info

Website title

Publisher / sponsor

URL

Electronically published

Williams, S. (2018, February 20). Serena Williams: What my life-threatening experience taught me about giving birth. CNN. https://www.cnn.com/2018/02/20/opinions/protect-mother-pregnancy-williams-opinion/index.html

_____

Glenda Hatchett on daughter-in-law's death: How does this happen?

TV Judge Glenda Hatchett and son push for greater maternal health care after loss of daughter-in-law. ... Their families came to California to celebrate the birth. In the end, they planned a funeral.

https://www.ajc.com/marketing/judge-glenda-hatchett-and-son-raise-awareness-maternal-....

Article title

TV Judge Glenda Hatchett and son fight for lives of new mothers

URL

https://www.ajc.com/marketing/judge-glenda-hatchett-and-son-raise-awareness-maternal-deaths/Z5Jg8DcqSz4NQLMKpP6PML/

Poole, S. M. (2018, March 9). TV judge Glenda Hatchett and Son Fight for lives of New Mothers. ajc. https://www.ajc.com/marketing/judge-glenda-hatchett-and-son-raise-awareness-maternal-deaths/Z5Jg8DcqSz4NQLMKpP6PML/

Website title ajc

Date accessed

May 28, 2023

Date published

March 09, 2018

Contributors

Position   First Name   MI / Middle   Last Name   Suffix

Add another contributor

Online publication info

Website title

Publisher / sponsor

URL   Electronically published   Day-?

—————

Death of Pregnant Black Woman, Sha-Asia Washington, Highlights Racial ...

The death of Sha-Asia Washington, a Black woman giving birth at a Brooklyn hospital, has prompted protests and petitions highlighting the racial disparities in maternal mortality in the U.S.

https://people.com/health/death-of-pregnant-black-woman-sha-asia-washington-highlights...

Article title

Death of Pregnant Black Woman, Sha-Asia Washington, Highlights Racial Disparities in Maternal Mortality

URL

https://people.com/health/death-of-pregnant-black-woman-sha-asia-washington-highlights-racial-disparities-in-maternal-mortality/

Website title Peoplemag

Date accessed

May 28, 2023

Date published

July 10, 2020

Mauch, A. (2020, July 10). Death of pregnant black woman, sha-asia washington, highlights racial disparities in maternal mortality. Peoplemag. https://people.com/health/death-of-pregnant-black-woman-sha-asia-washington-highlights-racial-disparities-in-maternal-mortality/

————

Beyoncé

Beyoncé Opens Up About Her Difficult Childbirth - The Cut

In the interview, Beyoncé discusses the historical significance of her cover, her performance at Coachella, and also opens up about her difficult pregnancy with her year-old twins, Rumi and Sir. "I was 218 pounds the day I gave birth to Rumi and Sir," she says, revealing that she was "swollen from toxemia," also known as preeclampsia ...

https://www.thecut.com/2018/08/beyonce-vogue-september-issue-twins-childbirth-c...

Article title

Beyoncé Opens Up About Her Difficult Pregnancy and Emergency C-Section

URL

https://www.thecut.com/2018/08/beyonce-vogue-september-issue-twins-childbirth-c-section.html

Website title The Cut

Date accessed

May 28, 2023

Date published

August 06, 2018

Aggeler, M. (2018, August 6). Beyoncé opens up about her difficult pregnancy and emergency C-section. The Cut. https://www.thecut.com/2018/08/beyonce-vogue-september-issue-twins-childbirth-c-section.html

—————-

Allyson Felix Opened up About Her Traumatic Birth at 32 Weeks - Insider

Olympian Allyson Felix made headlines when she broke Usain Bolt's gold-medal record just 10 months after giving birth via emergency C-section. Her gold-medal performance at the 2019 World Athletics Championships was impressive, but Felix later revealed that she felt pressured to return to the track as soon as possible because of her contract with her former sponsor, Nike.

https://www.insider.com/allyson-felix-opened-up-about-her-traumatic-birth-2021-12

Article title

Olympian Allyson Felix recalls the scariest day of her life. It was the day she gave birth.

URL

https://www.insider.com/allyson-felix-opened-up-about-her-traumatic-birth-2021-12

Website title Insider

Date accessed

May 28, 2023

Date published

December 16, 2021

Marcoux, H. (2021, December 16). Olympian Allyson Felix recalls the scariest day of her life. it was the day she gave birth. Insider. https://www.insider.com/allyson-felix-opened-up-about-her-traumatic-birth-2021-12

—————-

Amniocentesis: Purpose, Procedure, Risks, Recovery & Results

Amniocentesis is a prenatal test that can diagnose genetic disorders (such as Down syndrome and spina bifida) and other health issues in a fetus. A provider uses a needle to remove a small amount of amniotic fluid from inside your uterus, and then a lab tests the sample for specific conditions. Appointments & Access.

https://my.clevelandclinic.org/health/treatments/4206

Article title

Amniocentesis: Purpose, Procedure, Risks, Recovery & Results

URL

https://my.clevelandclinic.org/health/treatments/4206-genetic-amniocentesis

Website title Cleveland Clinic

professional, C. C. medical. (n.d.). Amniocentesis: Purpose, procedure, risks, Recovery & Results. Cleveland Clinic. https://my.clevelandclinic.org/health/treatments/4206-genetic-amniocentesis

—————

Date accessed

May 28, 2023

professional, C. C. medical. (n.d.). Amniocentesis: Purpose, procedure, risks, Recovery & Results. Cleveland Clinic. https://my.clevelandclinic.org/health/treatments/4206-genetic-amniocentesis)

Products. Cook Medical. (2021, May 13). https://www.cookmedical.com/products/wh_dan_webds/

—————

Article title

Products

URL

https://www.cookmedical.com/products/wh_dan_webds/

Website title Cook Medical

Date accessed

May 28, 2023

Date published

May 13, 2021

Disposable EchoTip® Amniocentesis Needle | Cook Medical

Disposable EchoTip® Amniocentesis Needle. Used for aspiration of fluid from the amniotic sac. EchoTip technology enhances the visualization of the needle tip under ultrasound. Needles with a distal sideport aid in fluid aspiration if the needle becomes clogged with debris. The products on this website are available for sale in the United States.

https://www.cookmedical.com/products/wh_dan_webds

————————

Mag sulf

Magnesium Sulfate and Premature Labor - Verywell Family

Magnesium sulfate is a tocolytic that has been used to slow or stop premature labor. Research shows that mag, like other tocolytics, doesn't work very well to actually prevent preterm birth, but it may help stall labor for a short time. Doctors may treat preterm labor with 48 hours of magnesium sulfate, hoping to buy enough time to complete a ...

https://www.verywellfamily.com/magnesium-sulfate-in-preterm-labor-2748458

Article title

Magnesium Sulfate and Premature Labor

URL

https://www.verywellfamily.com/magnesium-sulfate-in-preterm-labor-2748458

Website title

Verywell Family

Date accessed

May 28, 2023

Date published

June 14, 2021

Cheryl Bird, R. (2021, June 14). Magnesium sulfate and premature labor. Verywell Family. https://www.verywellfamily.com/magnesium-sulfate-in-preterm-labor-2748458

By Cheryl Bird, RN, BSN Updated on June 14, 2021

Medically reviewed by Meredith Shur, MD

Print

Magnesium sulfate, or mag for short, is used in pregnancy to prevent seizures due to worsening preeclampsia, to slow or stop preterm labor, and to prevent injuries to a preterm baby's brain.

Magnesium sulfate is given as an intravenous infusion or intramuscular injection in the hospital over 12 to 48 hours. It relaxes smooth muscle tissues, which helps to prevent seizures and slow uterine contractions.

Verywell / Alexandra Gordon

Uses

Magnesium sulfate infusions have been a common practice on obstetrical floors for more than 60 years. It's a well-studied drug, so doctors know very well how it affects moms and babies. Here is how it is used:

In Preterm Labor: To Allow Time For Steroids

Magnesium sulfate is a tocolytic that has been used to slow or stop premature labor. Research shows that mag, like other tocolytics, doesn't work very well to actually prevent preterm birth, but it may help stall labor for a short time.

Doctors may treat preterm labor with 48 hours of magnesium sulfate, hoping to buy enough time to complete a course of steroids to help the baby's lungs develop.

In Preeclampsia: To Prevent Seizures

Preeclampsia is a common complication of pregnancy that causes high blood pressure and protein in the urine. If not treated, preeclampsia can develop into eclampsia, a seizure disorder.

The only cure for preeclampsia and eclampsia is delivery of the baby, but magnesium sulfate can help prevent seizures in women with severe preeclampsia.

In Preterm Babies: To Protect Newborn Brains

Premature babies, especially those who are born before about 32 weeks gestation, have immature brains at birth. As they grow, they are at risk for cerebral palsy, a disorder that affects movement and intelligence.

Short-term (24 hours or less) infusions of magnesium sulfate have been shown to help protect the baby's brain by reducing the incidence of cerebral palsy.

Possible Side Effects

Magnesium sulfate infusion is safe and effective when administered for up to a week. However, its side effects can be very uncomfortable. In mothers, the side effects include:

Flushing or hot flashes

Feeling tired and lethargic

Nausea and vomiting

Dizziness

Blurred vision

Muscle weakness

These side effects during labor may make vaginal delivery difficult resulting in a C-section. However, magnesium sulfate administration is also shown to reduce post-operative pain. In addition, women who were given magnesium sulfate may experience a delay in milk production by up to 10 days.

In rare cases, respiratory depression can occur. This can be reversed with a calcium infusion and is more common in women with kidney problems.

Side Effects in Babies

Magnesium sulfate crosses the placenta to the baby, and babies may experience side effects that include poor muscle tone and low Apgar scores. These side effects are usually gone in a day or so and don't cause long-term problems.

Mag should not be given for longer than seven days, as long-term mag therapy can cause low calcium in the baby's bones.

Sources

By Cheryl Bird, RN, BSN

Cheryl Bird, RN, BSN, is a registered nurse in a tertiary level neonatal intensive care unit at Mary Washington Hospital in Fredericksburg, Virginia.

Cheryl Bird, R. (2021, June 14). Magnesium sulfate and premature labor. Verywell Family. https://www.verywellfamily.com/magnesium-sulfate-in-preterm-labor-2748458

—————-

Why steroids are recommended for preterm labor - BabyCenter

Your doctor may recommend the treatment if you're having symptoms of preterm labor, for example, or if you've been admitted to the hospital for a condition that may (or is scheduled to) result in an early delivery, such as preterm premature rupture of membranes (PPROM), cholestasis of pregnancy, or early preeclampsia.. Antenatal corticosteroids include the medications betamethasone (Celestone …

Article title

Betamethasone in pregnancy: How steroid shots can help your baby's lungs

URL

https://www.babycenter.com/pregnancy/your-body/should-i-take-steroids-during-preterm-labor_5437

Website title BabyCenter

Date accessed

May 28, 2023

Steroid shots help speed up the development of your baby's lungs, & Miles, K. (n.d.). Betamethasone in pregnancy: How steroid shots can help your baby's lungs. BabyCenter. https://www.babycenter.com/pregnancy/your-body/should-i-take-steroids-during-preterm-labor_5437

Fibroids

Article title

It's Not Normal: Black Women, Stop Suffering From Fibroids

URL

https://bwhi.org/2019/04/03/its-not-normal-black-women-stop-suffering-from-fibroids/

Website title Black Women's Health Imperative

Date accessed

May 28, 2023

Date published

April 03, 2019

https://bwhi.org/2019/04/03/its-not-normal-black-women-stop-suffering-from-fibroids/

It's Not Normal: Black Women, Stop Suffering From Fibroids

However, too many black women do not have an accurate idea of what normal really is. Women suffer needlessly before seeking treatment for their fibroids. The previously mentioned national survey showed that black women waited substantially longer than white women before seeking treatment – 4.5 years compared with 3.3 years.

https://bwhi.org/2019/04/03/its-not-normal-black

Article title

It's Not Normal: Black Women, Stop Suffering From Fibroids

URL

https://www.healthywomen.org/content/article/its-not-normal-black-women-stop-suffering-fibroids

Website title HealthyWomen

Date accessed

May 28, 2023

Date published

June 22, 2022

Editors, H. (2022, June 22). It's not normal: Black women, stop suffering from fibroids. HealthyWomen. https://www.healthywomen.org/content/article/its-not-normal-black-women-stop-suffering-fibroids

———

The United States Government. (2023, April 10). A proclamation on Black Maternal Health Week, 2023. The White House. https://www.whitehouse.gov/briefing-room/presidential-actions/2023/04/10/a-proclamation-on-black-maternal-health-week-2023/

———

https://www.mayoclinic.org/tests-procedures/anesthesia/about/pac-20384568

General anesthesia - Mayo Clinic. (2023, February 16).

————

https://www.mayoclinic.org/tests-procedures/anesthesia/about/pac-20384568

YouTube. (2019). *Closing the maternal mortality gap & improving outcomes for mothers. YouTube.* Retrieved June 1, 2023, from https://www.youtube.com/watch?v=kMZlfC0297s&t=10s.

TIMES LEADER `20/20' Transcript Reveals Patients' Stories Of Pain The Following Is A Transcript Of The Sept. 11 "20/20" Show About Former Hazleton-st. Joseph Medical Center Dr. Frank Ruhl Peterson, Who Pleaded Guilty To Charges That He Took Drugs Intended For Patients While He Worked At The Hospital And Conyngham Anesthesia Associates.

The following is a transcript of the Sept. 11 "20/20" show about former Hazleton-St. Joseph Medical Center Dr. Frank Ruhl Peterson, who pleaded guilty to charges that he took drugs intended for patients while he worked at the hospital and Conyngham Anesthesia AssociatesThe portion of the program was called, "Stealing relief. Doctor kept anesthesia for himself."

BARBARA WALTERS: Imagine that you are on an operating table, ready for surgery. You believe you've been given painkillers and you won't feel a thing. But then suddenly, a horrible shock, excruciating pain. You feel the knife as the surgeon cuts into you.

HUGH DOWNS: It happened exactly that way to some of the people you're going to meet in our first story tonight. The anesthesiologist was a drug abuser, and he was skimming the painkilling narcotics for himself.

Tom Jarriel has the bizarre tale of the doctor who became his patients' worst nightmare.

TOM JARRIEL: In the town of Hazleton in central Pennsylvania, people in need of medical care come to the top of the hill on Church Street, to Hazleton-St. Joseph Medical Center, fondly known as St. Joe's.

That's where Laurie Opiere went last summer when she needed major surgery to remove part of her colon. She expected discomfort, but not agony.

LAURIE OPIERE, SURGERY VICTIM: The worst memory that I have is that night. I can't describe it any differently.

JARRIEL: When Laurie awoke from surgery, she says she felt like she had been shot in the stomach.

LAURIE OPIERE: Tears started to come down my eyes. The pain was- it was horrible. It was the worst pain I've ever had in my life. And I couldn't tell anybody about it. I had a tube down my nose and I'm thinking, I have to tell somebody I'm in all this pain and I can't talk. What am I going to do?

JARRIEL: She says her anesthesiologist worked on her, but it didn't seem to help. She was left alone for the night.

LAURIE OPIERE: I had a needle in my spine and I was laying flat on my back. My legs were numb. I couldn't move my legs. My stomach had just been cut wide open and stapled back together. It's almost as if I was shot and left to die. That's what it felt like to me.

JARRIEL: Hours later, Dr. Donna Umale, another anesthesiologist, arrived on duty and says she heard cries of distress from Laurie's room.

DR. DONNA UMALE, ANESTHESIOLOGIST: Shout, shouting. I was in the nurse's station, and that is- her room is at the end of the hallway.

JARRIEL: Dr. Umale investigated.

DR. UMALE: I saw her doubling up in bed, sweaty, pale, and I said, "What's going on here?" The nurse told me, "There's no pain relief here." I said, "Did you tell Dr. Peterson? We cannot find him."

JARRIEL: Dr. Frank Peterson was Laurie's anesthesiologist, whose job it was to control her pain. He says he did. But Peterson had a secret. He was a drug addict, a man hiding a long criminal history with arrests for hitting a bus window with a steel bar; stealing money from a restaurant, an ex-heroin addict whose roots were in the tough streets of New York City.

He had been a taxi driver, an amateur boxer who earned a medical degree and believed he had kicked the drug habit. But he could only land a job on the Pacific island of American Samoa. There, he claims, an ankle injury led to painkillers and then more serious drugs- drugs found at the pharmacy in his new job at St. Joe's, drugs intended for patients like Sharon Kachmar.

SHARON KACHMAR, SURGERY VICTIM: Burning, pulling, just terrible, terrible pain.

JARRIEL: Sharon came to St. Joe's for a Caesarean section to deliver her son, Josh. Dr. Peterson gave her an epidural that was supposed to numb her from the waist down, but when the surgeon began cutting, Sharon says she felt the knife slicing into her skin.

SHARON KACHMAR: I screamed out and I yelled, "Wait a minute, I felt that." And Dr. Peterson said to me, "Well, don't mistake pressure for pain." And I said to him, this was not pressure, this was a sharp pain, a sharp cut.

JARRIEL: The greatest pain, she says, came when they reached into her womb to get the baby. She couldn't scream because Dr. Peterson was holding a mask to her face. Instead, she clutched her husband's hand.

SHARON KACHMAR: It felt like they were pulling my insides out, and I could feel myself being literally lifted off the table.

MR. KACHMAR, HUSBAND OF SHARON KACHMAR: I said to him, "Why is she squeezing my hand so hard? Is she feeling this?" And he looked at me and he said, "It's love, man, it's pure love." And he laughed.

JARRIEL: We found Dr. Frank Peterson in block 3C-1 of the Luzerne County Prison, convicted of burglary, drug possession and, most shocking of all, withholding drugs from his patients and using them himself.

Hospital records show how he did it. Peterson signed out massive amounts of a painkiller, a powerful narcotic, sufenta. On charts he wrote, he was giving it to his patients to relieve their pain. But instead, he diluted their doses and kept most of the sufenta for himself, leaving them in agony.

DR. FRANK PETERSON, CONVICTED ANESTHESIOLOGIST: Good morning.

JARRIEL: When Peterson spoke to us, he was a man without remorse for the treatment he had given his patients, regretting only that he had given doctors a bad name.

(interviewing) Each of these patients came with total faith that the system was going to provide them a doctor who had no problems who could handle their pain.

DR. PETERSON: Yes, and in that …

JARRIEL: And they feel it failed.

DR. PETERSON: And perhaps it did. I am not claiming innocence. I did something that was- it was terrible. I undermined the confidence of the public in the medical community. And that's- that can't be tolerated.

JARRIEL: (on camera) So how could this have happened? And should one man receive all the blame in a hospital with checks and balances to avoid just such a scandal?

Top administrators at St. Joe's hospital knew Peterson had a history of drug addiction when he started working there last June. But he told them he was clean, and they believe him. We wanted to ask the hospital how they could give staff privileges to a former drug addict and not keep close tabs on him. But they refused to speak with "20/20," citing pending litigation.

(voice over) In court documents, they've said they're the victims in this case. They were lied to by Peterson and acted reasonably and in an appropriate manner.

(interviewing) They say they were the victims of this, the hospital.

MARGARET KULKALSKI, FORMER NURSE SUPERVISOR, ST. JOSEPH'S HOSPITAL: No, the patients were the victims. The hospital? Once they knew that there was something wrong, then they were no longer the victims.

JARRIEL: (Voice over) Margaret Kulkalski was a nurse supervisor at St. Joe's, who has since been fired. She says she knows the hospital knew something was wrong because she went to management and told them that Peterson's procedures weren't working. His behavior was abnormal. The staff suspected he was using drugs.

Records "20/20" has obtained show Peterson was tested for drugs the very next day. Early results showed methadone, a class-2 illegal narcotic, in Peterson's urine. But surprisingly, he was not suspended. Eleven days later, he treated Laurie Opiere.

LAURIE OPIERE: I should never have been subjected to Dr. Peterson. He should not have been putting needles in people's spines. This never should have happened to me.

DR. PETERSON: The hospital did nothing wrong.

JARRIEL: (interviewing) Did nothing wrong?

DR. PETERSON: No, they did nothing wrong.

JARRIEL: They hire you, as a man who has an admitted record of addiction? They don't have close supervision …

DR. PETERSON: Is that a crime?

JARRIEL: Absolutely not. Except it's a good …

DR. PETERSON: Tom, Tom, my self-esteem is in your hands.

JARRIEL: … it's a good warning sign, something that perhaps they should have caught sooner than two months, it seems to me.

DR. PETERSON: A hospital is in a very delicate situation with this, and I can see where they were coming from.

JARRIEL: (voice over) Maybe Peterson can see where the hospital is coming from because he and they are now co-defendants in a malpractice lawsuit filed by Peterson's patients. Despite the fact that Peterson pled guilty to assaulting his patients by stealing their drugs, he now says he didn't do it. He claims he just took what was left over and did not cause patients needless pain.

(interviewing) Are you saying, Doctor, it was a strange coincidence that a number of patients, your patients, say they experienced extreme pain?

DR. PETERSON: That's something that I really can't answer.

JARRIEL: Your job was to control the pain.

DR. PETERSON: Well, first of all, you have to understand that pain is extremely subjective.

SHARON KACHMAR: I don't understand now …

JARRIEL: (voice over) Tell that to these people. They say Dr. Peterson's procedures left them in excruciating pain during what was supposed to be a time of joy- childbirth.

1ST FEMALE SURGERY VICTIM ON PANEL: I felt everything. I felt all that pain because of him.

2ND FEMALE SURGERY VICTIM ON PANEL: How he can say he didn't cause pain when he knew consciously that he was skimping on medication …

HUSBAND OF VICTIM JILL POPOLIS: Yes, he definitely did not care, because while Jill was complaining about being in pain, he sat behind her and was flipping through the pages of a novel.

SHARON KACHMAR: I just don't understand how a human being who is supposed to be a doctor can do something like that.

DR. UMALE: As a physician, I think patients should be protected.

JARRIEL: (interviewing) Were Dr. Peterson's patients being protected?

DR. UMALE: I don't think they were protected, because they suffered.

JARRIEL: Dr. Umale says she was so angry at hospital administrators for allowing Peterson to continue, she decided to resign. Incredibly, there was talk of giving Peterson a promotion. Then something even more amazing happened- the hospital received final test results, proof that Peterson was using sufenta, the narcotic he was supposed to be giving his patients.

But still he was allowed to continue his work unsupervised. The next day, it took Peterson four tries to insert an epidural needle into Jill Popolis' back to prepare her for a C-section. When the operation began, she says she felt the surgeon's knife.

JILL POPOLIS, SURGERY VICTIM: And Dr. Peterson commented that, "Oh, no. You didn't feel anything. You didn't feel that."

JARRIEL: (interviewing) You went through terrible pain from a man who had just failed a drug test.

JILL POPOLIS: I couldn't believe that I put my trust into all those doctors and that hospital, and they will let someone like that work on a patient.

HUSBAND OF JILL POPOLIS: Total shock. Total shock.

JARRIEL: They say you were their worst nightmare. That they came to you to relieve their pain during a moment of crisis in their lives, and the pain was not relieved.

DR. PETERSON: Well, I can just answer your question with a question. What did they do before the invention of epidurals? Somehow we've made it through several million years of childbirth. It's amazing we're still here, isn't it?

JARRIEL: (voice over) Finally, on Aug. 8th, two months and five days after he began, St. Joe's hospital suspended Frank Peterson. But they didn't call the police until four days later, after he broke into the hospital and stole more drugs.

Ed Harry was the detective who investigated the case, turning up a large cache of drugs and paraphernalia in Peterson's home.

(on camera) Whoa, looks like he was running a hospital.

ED HARRY, DETECTIVE: All of the rooms that we went into had catheters, needles, hypodermic syringes, IV tubing, empty vials of drugs.

JARRIEL: (voice over) Harry says Peterson made a full confession.

ED HARRY: I asked him how many of the patients that he had did he take drugs from?

JARRIEL: (interviewing) Right.

ED HARRY: And he said, "All of them."

JARRIEL: Did he express any sorrow, any sympathy, any empathy at all for the patients that he had put through this pain?

ED HARRY: No, he didn't. His main concern was losing his medical license.

JARRIEL: Peterson has lost that license to practice medicine in Pennsylvania for 10 years. But like the boxer he once was, Peterson may be down, but he's not out of the medical profession.

DR. PETERSON: There are possibilities that I can go overseas. There are some countries who desperately need physicians who aren't encumbered by the morass of legality that this country is. They say a fool is one who does not learn from experience. I've been pretty much of a fool so far. Let's hope I can wise up.

BARBARA WALTERS: Mmm! Can you just imagine his former patients? Well, Frank Peterson is now out of prison. He is attending a drug treatment program, and Hugh, he is working as a cook.

HUGH DOWNS: I'd want to be on a diet, I think.-

ABC News, "20/20"

OBTAINING MEDICAL RECORDS, REPORT AND INCIDENT REPORTS

TOOL KIT:

- copies of the medical records of treatment
- copies of medical reports of medical examination/surgical performance

   a. Medical record is just a **record** of the patient's medical/operative treatment while in the hospital.
   b. Medical report a **report** of a medical examination or surgical performance
   c. Incident reports are an **internal** tool used to document issues and are **NOT** part of the medical record.

Processes involved and the necessary Precautionary Measures

- Be specific about record request or range of dates, day or year.
- Use a broader range if the actual date is not sure of.
- When the actual date is not sure of, use a broader range even if it overlaps the day in question. Otherwise, the individual's request will come back with a responding note, stating, "no record(s) found".
- Having knowledge of Freedom of Information Law (FOIL and the Freedom of Information Acts (FOLA)

   a. Freedom Of Information Law (State, County, City and Local Municipalities)

- Differentiate between a **FOIL** and **FOIA**

   Everything You Need To Know About The Freedom Of Information Law The New York State Freedom of Information Law, outlined in Article 6 of the New York Public Officers Law, was enacted in 1974 to make government more transparent for New Yorkers.

   b. Freedom Of Information Act (Federal)

   The Freedom of Information Act, 5 U.S.C. § 552 § 552. Public information; agency rules, opinions, orders, records, and Proceedings (a) Each agency shall make available to the public information as follows: (1) Each agency shall separately state and currently publish in the Federal Register for the guidance of the public—

- To assure the safety of the original set of documents, always make photocopies before redacting any documents and store them somewhere separately.
- Redact all personal and confidential information that one wishes not to share or publicize including the names and exposure of Doctors and Nurses.
- Do not stack papers on top of one another because the marker will bleed through and destroy the content on the following pages. This is one of the most important and major reasons why one should always make duplicate copies first.
- Use a black permanent marker.
- Once redacted, make sure no one can not read or see through the blacked out coverage.
- It is possible the redaction may take a 2nd or 3rd marking before fully covered.
- Be careful when using markers and try not to make any unnecessary markings.
- Using the online patient portal to retrieve medical records.

When a medical record is received, be sure the photo copies don't overlap covering up pertinent information making it illegible. (See: enclosed copy on how one page partially covers up the others content); no one is sure what's covered up here. But I sure would have liked to have known!

Please note, when hospitalized, the patient is closely monitored and everything that is said or done will be documented and logged onto the patient chart.

Patient Compliance and Non Compliance:

- Sometimes it may be necessary and within one's rights to refuse, i.e., prevent possible early labor and contractions, due to the use of the TENs device that could cause electrical muscle stimulation to the fetus as well.
- The patient involved must make the choice depending on the better outcome for both her and her unborn baby complications, preterm labor, placental abruption and premature rupture of the membrane.

Patient Safety:

5 Tips of what a patient can do to Be a Safe Patient 5 Tips [Video – 2:32]

- Protect oneself and the family from harmful hands germs
- Regular hand cleaning is one of the best ways to remove germs
- Avoid getting sick, and prevent spreading germs
- Take antibiotics only when the provider thinks the patient needs them.
- Ask if an antibiotic is necessary.

Understanding a medical report:

- By placing the word medical after each word, abbreviation or letter
- one will then be able to find its definition
- therefore reference it
- cross match it back to your specific condition

FOIL LAW SIMPLIFY

Matt McLaughlin, partner-in-charge of Venable's New York office, is a commercial litigator who represents clients in complex commercial and securities matters, intellectual property and product liability disputes, and construction litigation, primarily in New York state and federal courts, and before arbitration and mediation panels. Matt has extensive experience in transnational litigation and in advising clients in the developing law related to electronic signatures. He also has extensive knowledge of the Freedom of Information Law (FOIL) and Freedom of Information Act (FOIA) statutes, having advised New York state, municipal, and quasi-governmental not-for-profit organizations responding to and defending against freedom of expression information requests.

Matt is also experienced in transnational litigation, including operation of the Hague Convention, and letters rogatory in the Swiss, Canadian, UK, German, and Norwegian courts. His work includes litigating mutual legal assistance treaty (MLAT) requests by foreign governments under 28 U.S.C. 1782. Matt has also coordinated parallel proceedings in a variety of non-U.S. jurisdictions.

https://www.venable.com/insights/publications/2022/08/foil-law-simplified

(DCD), D. C. D. (2023, April 20). How can I complain about poor medical care I received in a hospital?. HHS.gov. https://www.hhs.gov/answers/health-insurance-reform/how-can-i-complain-about-poor-medical-care/index.html

David Cruz Published Sep 11, 2021 Share Facebook Twitter Reddit Email, & James Ramsay Published Jun 2, 2023 at 2:09 p.m. (n.d.). *Everything you need to know about the freedom of information law.* Gothamist. https://gothamist.com/news/everything-you-need-know-freedom-of-information-law-foil-explainer.

FILING A COMPLAINT

- Always take someone to the hospital, or have someone on the phone listening in with permission to advocate for you if need be, just be sure to inform the Doctor while doing so.
- In the Doctor's office, if your complaint is not taken seriously, then tell your doctor to please note such in your chart, of what your stated illness is being refused and treated for.
- File a **QUALITY OF CARE** complaint with the Insurance Company.
- File a complaint with the **STATE MEDICAL BOARD.**
- File a complaint with the **HOSPITAL ADMINISTRATOR** whether on the phone or in person put the complaint in writing via email follow-up that way you have a digital trial. Also, because it is illegal to record someone without their consent. Therefore, if you happen to have a recording, then have someone type it out verbatim. Although, it's your word against theirs, but at least you have it.

PATIENT SAFETY

11 September 2023

العربية

中文

Français

Русский

Español

Key facts

- **Around 1 in every 10 patients is harmed in health care and more than 3 million deaths occur annually due to unsafe care. In low-to-middle income countries, as many as 4 in 100 people die from unsafe care (1).**
- **Above 50% of harm (1 in every 20 patients) is preventable; half of this harm is attributed to medications (2,3).**
- **Some estimates suggest that as many as 4 in 10 patients are harmed in primary and ambulatory settings, while up to 80% (23.6–85%) of this harm can be avoided (4).**
- **Common adverse events that may result in avoidable patient harm are medication errors, unsafe surgical procedures, health care-associated infections, diagnostic errors, patient falls, pressure ulcers, patient misidentification, unsafe blood transfusion and venous thromboembolism.**
- **Patient harm potentially reduces global economic growth by 0.7% a year. On a global scale, the indirect cost of harm amounts to trillions of US dollars each year (1).**
- **Investment in reducing patient harm can lead to significant financial savings, and more importantly better patient outcomes (5). An example of a good return on investment is patient engagement, which, if done well, can reduce the burden of harm by up to 15% (4).**

Overview

"First, do no harm" is the most fundamental principle of any health care service. No one should be harmed in health care; however, there is compelling evidence of a huge burden of avoidable patient harm globally across the developed and developing health care systems. This has major human, moral, ethical and financial implications.

Patient safety is defined as "the absence of preventable harm to a patient and reduction of risk of unnecessary harm associated with health care to an acceptable minimum." Within the broader health system context, it is "a framework of organized activities that creates cultures, processes, procedures, behaviours, technologies and environments in health care that consistently and sustainably lower risks, reduce the occurrence of avoidable harm, make error less likely and reduce impact of harm when it does occur."

Common sources of patient harm

Medication errors. Medication-related harm affects 1 out of every 30 patients in health care, with more than a quarter of this harm regarded as severe or life threatening. Half of the avoidable harm in health care is related to medications *(3)*.

Surgical errors. Over 300 million surgical procedures are performed each year worldwide *(6)*. Despite awareness of adverse effects, surgical errors continue to occur at a high rate; 10% of preventable patient harm in health care was reported in surgical settings *(2)*, with most of the resultant adverse events occurring pre- and post-surgery *(7)*.

Health care-associated infections. With a global rate of 0.14% (increasing by 0.06% each year), health care-associated infections result in extended duration of hospital stays, long-standing disability, increased antimicrobial resistance, additional financial burden on patients, families and health systems, and avoidable deaths *(8)*.

Sepsis. Sepsis is a serious condition that happens when the body's immune system has an extreme response to an infection. The body's reaction causes damage to its own tissues and organs. Of all sepsis cases managed in hospitals, 23.6% were found to be health care associated, and approximately 24.4% of affected patients lost their lives as a result *(9)*.

Diagnostic errors. These occur in 5–20% of physician–patient encounters *(10,11)*. According to doctor reviews, harmful diagnostic errors were found in a minimum of 0.7% of adult admissions *(12)*. Most people will suffer a diagnostic error in their lifetime *(13)*.

Patient falls. Patient falls are the most frequent adverse events in hospitals *(14)*. Their rate of occurrence ranges from 3 to 5 per 1000 bed-days, and more than one third of these incidents result in injury *(15)*, thereby reducing clinical outcomes and increasing the financial burden on systems *(16)*.

Venous thromboembolism. More simply known as blood clots, venous thromboembolism is a highly burdensome and preventable cause of patient harm, which contributes to one third of the complications attributed to hospitalization *(17)*.

Pressure ulcers. Pressure ulcers are injuries to the skin or soft tissue. They develop from pressure to particular parts of the body over an extended period. If not promptly managed, they can have fatal complications. Pressure ulcers affect more than 1 in 10 adult patients admitted to hospitals *(18)* and, despite being highly preventable, they have a significant impact on the mental and physical health of individuals, and their quality of life.

Unsafe transfusion practices. Unnecessary transfusions and unsafe transfusion practices expose patients to the risk of serious adverse transfusion reactions and transfusion-transmissible infections. Data on adverse transfusion reactions from a group of 62 countries show an average incidence of 12.2 serious reactions per 100 000 distributed blood components.

Patient misidentification. Failure to correctly identify patients can be a root cause of many problems and has serious effects on health care provision. It can lead to catastrophic adverse effects, such as wrong-site surgery. A report of the Joint Commission published in 2018 identified 409 sentinel events of patient identification out of 3326 incidents (12.3%) between 2014 and 2017 *(19)*.

Unsafe injection practices. Each year, 16 billion injections are administered worldwide, and unsafe injection practices place patients and health and care workers at risk of infectious and non-infectious adverse events. Using mathematical modelling, a study estimated that, in a period of 10 years (2000–2010), 1.67 million hepatitis B virus infections, between 157 592 and 315 120 hepatitis C virus infections, and between 16 939 and 33 877 HIV infections were associated with unsafe injections *(20)*.

Factors leading to patient harm

Patient harm in health care due to safety breaks is pervasive, problematic and can occur in all settings and at all levels of health care provision. There are multiple and interrelated factors that can lead to patient harm, and more than one factor is usually involved in any single patient safety incident:

- system and organizational factors: the complexity of medical interventions, inadequate processes and procedures, disruptions in workflow and care coordination, resource constraints, inadequate staffing and competency development;
- technological factors: issues related to health information systems, such as problems with electronic health records or medication administration systems, and misuse of technology;
- human factors and behaviour: communication breakdown among health care workers, within health care teams, and with patients and their families, ineffective teamwork, fatigue, burnout, and cognitive bias;
- patient-related factors: limited health literacy, lack of engagement and non-adherence to treatment; and
- external factors: absence of policies, inconsistent regulations, economic and financial pressures, and challenges related to natural environment.

System approach to patient safety

Most of the mistakes that lead to harm do not occur as a result of the practices of one or a group of health and care workers but are rather due to system or process failures that lead these health and care workers to make mistakes.

Understanding the underlying causes of errors in medical care thus requires shifting from the traditional blaming approach to a more system-based thinking. In this, errors are attributed to poorly designed system structures and processes, and the human nature of all those working in health care facilities under a considerable amount of stress in complex and quickly changing environments is recognized. This is done without overlooking negligence or misbehaviour from those providing care that leads to substandard medical management.

A safe health system is one that adopts all necessary measures to avoid and reduce harm through organized activities, including:

- ensuring leadership commitment to safety and creation of a culture whereby safety is prioritized;
- ensuring a safe working environment and the safety of procedures and clinical processes;
- building competencies of health and care workers and improving teamwork and communication;
- engaging patients and families in policy development, research and shared decision-making; and
- establishing systems for patient safety incident reporting for learning and continuous improvement.

Investing in patient safety positively impacts health outcomes, reduces costs related to patient harm, improves system efficiency, and helps in reassuring communities and restoring their trust in health care systems *(4,5)*.

WHO response

Global action on patient safety

Recognizing patient safety as a global health priority, and as an essential component of strengthening health systems for moving towards universal health coverage, the Seventy-second World Health Assembly adopted resolution WHA72.6 on "Global action on patient safety" in May 2019.

The resolution requested the Director-General to emphasize patient safety as a key strategic priority in WHO's work across the universal health coverage agenda, endorsed the establishment of World Patient Safety Day to be observed annually on 17 September, and requested WHO's Director-General to develop a global patient safety action plan with the involvement of WHO Member States, partners and other relevant stakeholders.

Global Patient Safety Action Plan 2021–2030

The Global Patient Safety Action Plan 2021–2030 provides a framework for action for key stakeholders to join efforts and implement patient safety initiatives in a comprehensive manner. The goal is "to achieve the maximum possible reduction in avoidable harm due to unsafe health care globally", envisioning "a world in which no one is harmed in health care, and every patient receives safe and respectful care, every time, everywhere".

World Patient Safety Day

Since 2019, World Patient Safety Day has been celebrated across the world annually on 17 September, calling for global solidarity and concerted action by all countries and international partners to improve patient safety. The global campaign, with its dedicated annual theme, is aimed at enhancing public awareness and global understanding of patient safety and mobilizing action by stakeholders to eliminate avoidable harm in health care and thereby improve patient safety.

WHO has launched the Patient Safety Flagship as a transformative initiative to guide and support strategic action on patient safety at the global, regional and national levels. Its core work involves supporting the implementation of the Global Patient Safety Action Plan 2021–2030.

References

1. Slawomirski L, Klazinga N. The economics of patient safety: from analysis to action. Paris: Organisation for Economic Co-operation and Development; 2020 (http://www.oecd.org/health/health-systems/Economics-of-Patient-Safety-October-2020.pdf, accessed 6 September 2023).

2. Panagioti M, Khan K, Keers RN, Abuzour A, Phipps D, Kontopantelis E et al. Prevalence, severity, and nature of preventable patient harm across medical care settings: systematic review and meta-analysis. BMJ. 2019;366:l4185. doi:10.1136/bmj.l4185.

3. Hodkinson A, Tyler N, Ashcroft DM, Keers RN, Khan K, Phipps D et al. Preventable medication harm across health care settings: a systematic review and meta-analysis. BMC Med. 2020;18(1):1–3.

4. Slawomirski L, Auraaen A, Klazinga N. The economics of patient safety in primary and ambulatory care: flying blind. OECD Health Working Papers No. 106. Paris: Organisation for Economic Co-operation and Development; 2018 (https://doi.org/10.1787/baf425ad-en, accessed 6 September 2023).

5. Slawomirski L, Auraaen A, Klazinga N. The economics of patient safety: strengthening a value-based approach to reducing patient harm at national level. OECD Health Working Papers No. 96. Paris: Organisation for Economic Co operation and Development; 2017 (https://doi.org/10.1787/5a9858cd-en, accessed 6 September 2023).

6. Meara, John G., Andrew JM Leather, Lars Hagander, Blake C. Alkire, Nivaldo Alonso, Emmanuel A. Ameh, et al. Global Surgery 2030: evidence and solutions for achieving health, welfare, and economic development. The lancet. 2015; 386: 569-624

7. Rodziewicz TL, Houseman B, Hipskind JE. Medical error reduction and prevention. Treasure Island, FL: StatPearls Publishing; 2023.

8. Raoofi S, Kan FP, Rafiei S, Hosseinipalangi Z, Mejareh ZN, Khani S et al. Global prevalence of nosocomial infection: a systematic review and meta-analysis. PLoS One. 2023;18(1):e0274248.

9. Markwart R, Saito H, Harder T, Tomczyk S, Cassini A, Fleischmann-Struzek C et al. Epidemiology and burden of sepsis acquired in hospitals and intensive care units: a systematic review and meta-analysis. Intensive Care Med. 2020;46(8):1536–51. doi:10.1007/s00134-020-06106-2.

10. National Academies of Sciences, Engineering, and Medicine. Improving diagnosis in health care. Washington (DC): National Academies Press; 2015 (https://doi.org/10.7326/M15-2256, accessed 6 September 2023).

11. Bergl PA, Nanchal RS, Singh H. Diagnostic error in the critically ill: defining the problem and exploring next steps to advance intensive care unit safety. Ann Am Thorac Soc. 2018;15(8):903–7.

12. Gunderson CG, Bilan VP, Holleck JL, Nickerson P, Cherry BM, Chui P et al. Prevalence of harmful diagnostic errors in hospitalised adults: a systematic review and meta-analysis. BMJ Qual Saf. 2020;29(12):1008–18.

13. Singh H, Meyer AN, Thomas EJ. The frequency of diagnostic errors in outpatient care: estimations from three large observational studies involving US adult populations. BMJ Qual Saf. 2014;23(9):727–31.

14. LeLaurin JH, Shorr RI. Preventing falls in hospitalized patients: state of the science. Clin Geriatr Med. 2019;35(2):273–83.

15. Agency for Healthcare Research and Quality. Falls. PSNet; 2019. (https://psnet.ahrq.gov/primer/falls, accessed 11 September 2023).

16. Dykes PC, Curtin-Bowen M, Lipsitz S, Franz C, Adelman J, Adkison L et al. Cost of inpatient falls and cost-benefit analysis of implementation of an evidence-based fall prevention program. JAMA Health Forum. 2023;4(1):e225125. doi:10.1001/jamahealthforum.2022.5125.

17. Raskob GE, Angchaisuksiri P, Blanco AN, Buller H, Gallus A, Hunt BJ et al. Thrombosis: a major contributor to global disease burden. Arterioscler Thromb Vasc Biol. 2014;34(11):2363–71. doi:10.1161/ATVBAHA.114.304488.

18. Li Z, Lin F, Thalib L, Chaboyer W. Global prevalence and incidence of pressure injuries in hospitalised adult patients: A systematic review and meta-analysis. International journal of nursing studies. 2020 May 1;105:103546.

19. De Rezende HA, Melleiro MM, Shimoda GT. Interventions to reduce patient identification errors in the hospital setting: a systematic review protocol. JBI Evidence Synthesis. 2019;17(1):37–42.

20. Pèpin J, Chakra CN, Pèpin E, Nault V, Valiquette L. Evolution of the global burden of viral infections from unsafe medical injections, 2000-2010. PLoS One. 2014;9(6):e99677.

Related

- Global Patient Safety Action Plan 2021-2030
- The conceptual framework for the international classification for patient safety
- 10 facts on patient safety
- Global Ministerial Summits on Patient Safety
- World Patient Safety Day

News

Global stakeholders agree to a new charter on patient safety rights

14 September 2023

Fact sheets

Antimicrobial resistance

21 November 2023

Blood safety and availability

2 June 2023

Ionizing radiation and health effects

27 July 2023

Sepsis

19 July 2023

Universal health coverage (UHC)

5 October 2023

Events

Sixth Global Ministerial Summit on Patient Safety 2024 "Bringing and sustaining changes in patient safety policies and practices"

17 – 18 April 2024

1. Archives
2. 2009 Volume 6 Number 3 July- September
3. Patient Non-Compliance— A Powerful Legal Defense

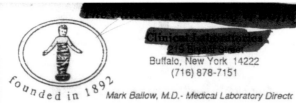

Clinical Laboratories
2/5 Bryant Street
Buffalo, New York 14222
(716) 878-7151

founded in 1892

Mark Ballow, M.D.- Medical Laboratory Director

HEMAT⊙

Collection Date:	03/09/97	03/08/97	03/07/97		
Collection Time:	0631	0000	1105		

-PROCEDURE-

HEMOGRAM

WBC x10^9/L	11.9 H	12.7 H	18.0 H	11.9 H	4...	
RBC x10	3.80 L	4.34	4.20	4.42	4.20-5.4	
HGB g/			12.2 L	12.8	12.5-16.0	
HCT %				- -	37.0-47.0	
MCV fL	85					
MCH pg	28					
MCHC g						
PLT x1						
RDW %						
MPV fl						
CBC C						

SERVICE ORDERED:

CHILDREN'S HOSPITAL OF BUFFALO

☒ PHYSICAL THERAPY   ☐ OCCUPATIONAL THERAPY

PATIENT NAME
Chillis Eleanore

UNIT NUMBER
V-5

TREATMENT NOTES ☒   DISCHARGE SUMMARY ☐

3/3/97 - 3/7/97 Pt is 40 y/o ♀ pregnant c̄ dx of mild pre-eclampsia
degenerative fibroids and c/o pain in Ⓑ groin area + wrists.
3/3/97 Pt rec'd wrist braces for pain in wrists when transferring.
Pt refused use of TENS unit. Pt Ⓘ in bed mob, transfers in + out
of bed and amb x20ft sliding both feet along floor. Pt
moved to 3rd floor on 3/6/97 + receiving med for ↑ BP. Did LE
ther ex. on 3/7/97. Pt non compliant in ther ex and may
deliver baby on 3/8/97 in am. Continue c̄ ther. ex. Plan to
modify ex. program s̄ baby is born as appropriate.
SPT/ _____ PT

COAGU

PT	
INR	
PTT	
FIBRINOGEN	412 H

Key:
L = Low, H = High
Key:
">" = Greater than, "<" = Less than, ">=" = Greater than or equal, "< " = Less than or equal

Patient: CHILLIS, ELEANOR E   Print: 3/14/1997 at 405
Admission Date: 02/27/1997   Page 1
Discharge Date: 03/12/1997   Continued...

F2054

...D OF STAY SUMMARY Not Di d

PATIENT NON-COMPLIANCE— A POWERFUL LEGAL DEFENSE

By: Becky Summey-Lowman, LD, CPHRM

This article is reprinted with permission from Healthcare Risk Manager, a publication of MAG Mutual Insurance Company's Risk Management/Patient Safety Department, Vol. 15, Number 1. There is little doubt to any practicing physician that patient non-compliance is a significant and contributory factor to poor outcomes. There is also little doubt that patient non-compliance can often lead to more aggressive and costly treatments. What you may not know is the extent that to which a patient's noncompliance can increase your risk for a medical malpractice claim and how much good documentation can protect you. While it is reasonable for you to expect a patient to share in the responsibility for their own care, juries nationwide have placed a significant amount of responsibility for follow-up on the provider. When patients fail to follow treatment advice, it is prudent to document this in the medical record. There are compelling reasons for providers to document patient noncompliance. If such non-compliance contributes to an injury that results in a malpractice suit, it can usually be introduced as evidence in the doctor's defense. Documentation of patient noncompliance can may provide a powerful defense to any lawsuit. Depending upon the comparative fault laws in your state, a plaintiff's recovery is reduced or prohibited based on the percentage fault attributed to the plaintiff. A recent case involved the death, while hospitalized, of a 39 year old 6'4, 225 white male 11 days post bilateral laminectomy and lumbar decompression at the L3-4 and L4-5 from a pulmonary embolism. The MAG Mutual insured neurosurgeon ordered TED and SCD devices for the patient upon his presentation in the emergency department. This order was never discontinued, but the patient was non-compliant throughout his hospitalization, despite repeated education by the medical team of the risk associated with a deep vein thrombosis (DVT). The plaintiff contended that because our physician never documented his conversation with the patient regarding the possible risk of DVT and because he failed to implement heparin therapy these actions rose to the level of malpractice. The MAG Mutual defense team put forth a strong defense that showed the patient's refusal to follow medical instructions and the risks associated with heparin therapy. Our physician did an excellent job during his testimony educating the jury about the surgical procedure including his normal practice of explaining the risks associated with blood clots. It was also brought out in the testimony by the nurses, physical therapist and nursing assistant regarding their diligence in ambulating the patient and explaining the risk for DVT to both the patient and his wife. After a week of trial the jury returned a defense verdict, following 45 minutes of deliberations. Non-Compliance versus Patient's Right to Make Decision Regarding Medical Treatments. It is important to recognize the difference between noncompliance and the patient's right to refuse care. Patients have the right to make informed decisions regarding their care, including being informed of their health status, being involved in care planning and treatment, and being able to request or refuse treatment. Non-compliance may be the result of an educated, rational and reasonable decision on the patient's part to exercise control over their healthcare. The medical record should include documentation that the diagnosis and proposed procedure/treatments were explained to the patient and that the explanation included the patient's prognosis without the procedure, the risks and benefits, and alternative therapies. Consider the following suggestions to enhance patient compliance:

- Emphasize the seriousness and urgency of any recommended tests.
- Explain the rationale for your treatment advice
- Allow the patient to voice any concerns they have about recommended treatments
- Suggest treatments that are reasonable, taking into account the patient's lifestyle, finances and ability to comply
- Whenever possible, give patients the opportunity to think about proposed treatments prior to making a final decision
- Provide simple written information to patients and others who are involved in their care
- Attempt to gain agreement on the treatment plan effective."

A sample informed refusal form can be found on the MAG Mutual website at www.magmutual.com. Risk Management Strategies Document Non-Compliance/Informed Refusal When the patient has failed to comply with your recommendations, document the non-compliance. Among the more common problem areas are:

- Repeated failure to keep appointments;
- Failure to have diagnostic testing or consultation as recommended
- Failure to comply with medication therapy
- Failure to follow medication monitoring recommendations (for example, warfarin monitoring)

Carefully notate episodes of non-compliance, avoiding any documentation that may look judgmental or self-serving. An example of an adequately documented informed refusal discussion is as follows: "A breast ultrasound has been recommended to evaluate the palpable lesion on the right breast. The patient states that her insurance "will not be effective for ninety days" and elects not to have the test done pending coverage by insurance plan. The risk of delay was discussed with the patient to include the possibility of a malignancy, and the risks of a potentially life threatening delay in diagnosis and treatment. The patient verbalizes understanding of the information provided. I have asked my staff to investigate and advise her of any financial assistance that may be available. She was advised to contact me as soon as possible if she reconsiders this decision or as soon as insurance coverage is Document Screening Recommendations Advise patients of preventative health screenings and document these discussions. Failure to do so could result in an allegation of a delay in diagnosis if a metastatic or potentially life-threatening condition is not detected in a timely manner. Inform Patients of Test Results in a Timely Manner Inform patients of test results in a timely manner. Results that are indicative of a potentially life threatening illness may be best communicated by the physician personally to allow the patient the opportunity for questions and agreement on future treatment plans. Maintain a Reliable Clinical Tracking System Without a reliable clinical tracking system, it may be difficult to identify patients who fail to keep scheduled appointments for tests and consultations with specialists. Whenever possible, schedule referrals and follow-up appointments before the patient leave the office. If the patient refuses the test, due to financial or other reasons, this should be well documented. Failure to maintain reliable clinical tracking systems is one of the most frequently cited problems in medical malpractice cases where there is an allegation of delay in diagnosis and/or failure to supervise care. Coordinate Treatment Plans with Other Providers Involved in the Patient's Care Maintain good communication with other providers involved in the patient's care and maintain a clear understanding of the expectations and role in the patient's plan of care. Ask consultants to notify you if the patient fails to keep an appointment and request periodic updates on the care and treatment plan or a summary at the conclusion of care, whichever is appropriate. Informed Consent Inform patients regarding any alternatives, benefits, risks and complications associated with the proposed treatments or tests. Document all informed consent and informed refusal discussions. In conclusion, given the extensive research on patient noncompliance, it is reasonable to maintain a high index of suspicion for non-compliance on all patients. The best approach is to maintain effective communications with patients and take proactive measures to enhance treatment goals. However, when patients fail to follow recommended advice and a poor outcomes result in a medical malpractice claim, objective documentation of non-compliance can be your most powerful defense. References: 1. The Food and Drug Administration and the National Council on Patient Information. Healthy Living: Be a Good Patient and Follow Directions. Available at www.healthlink. com/health_good_patient.asp. Accessed 30 Sept. 2003. 2. The Prevalence and Incidence of Patient Noncompliance Section, with citations, is available for download in PDF format from Dr. Showalter's Align- Map.com site: ~Noncompliance Incidence and Prevalence~ 3. Online Reference http://www. musc.edu/catalyst/ archive/2001/co1-19pharmacy.htm 04/02/01,11785 bytes

Self-Insurance Programs
Copyright© 2024

HOW CAN I COMPLAIN ABOUT POOR MEDICAL CARE I RECEIVED IN A HOSPITAL?

While you're in the hospital:

Bring your complaints to your doctor and nurses as soon as possible. Be as specific as you can and ask how your complaint can be resolved. You can also ask to speak to a hospital social worker who can help solve problems and identify resources. Social workers also organize services and paperwork when patients leave the hospital.

Contact your state's <u>Beneficiary and Family Centered Care Quality Improvement Organization (BFCC-QIO)</u> for complaints about the quality of care you got from a Medicare provider.

You can submit a complaint to your BFCC-QIO for things like getting the wrong medication, having the wrong surgery or treatment, or getting discharged too early. <u>Learn more about filing a complaint on Medicare.gov</u>.

You can also find your BFCC-QIO by calling 1-800-MEDICARE (1-800-633-4227). TTY users can call 1-877-468-2048.

If you get an infection while you're in the hospital or have problems getting the right medication, you can file a complaint with the <u>Joint Commission</u> . This group certifies many U.S. hospitals' safety and security practices and investigates complaints about patients' rights. It does not oversee medical care or how the hospital may bill you.

<u>Visit Medicare.gov to find survey ratings</u> from hospital patients about their care. You can compare information about a hospital's performance against national averages for patient experiences, timely and effective care, complications, and more.

If you're discharged before you're ready:

This is a big concern for many patients because sometimes insurers don't approve long hospital stays. Talk to the hospital discharge planner (often a social worker) if you don't think you're medically ready to leave the hospital. The discharge planner will take your concerns to the doctor who makes this decision.

If you're covered by Medicare or by a Medicare-managed care plan, you can file an appeal about a discharge while you're still in the hospital. You should get a form from the hospital titled "An Important Message from Medicare," which explains how to appeal a hospital discharge decision. Appeals are free and generally resolved in two to three days. The hospital cannot discharge you until the appeal is completed. Learn more about Medicare appeals.

If you don't agree with your hospital bill:

First, ask your doctor or the hospital's billing department to explain the charges. Then, find out how the hospital handles complaints about bills and make your case. Changes to federal law may help protect you from surprise medical bills and allow you to dispute your bill. If you have Medicare and you don't agree with your bill, you can file an appeal.

You can also call 1-800-MEDICARE about billing questions. Make sure you have the date of service, the total charge in question, and the name of your doctor and hospital. TTY users can call 1-877-468-2048

Even with this information, it isn't easy to be as assertive in a health care setting as it is in an auto repair shop or restaurant. But it's a smart move that can help you get the quality care that you deserve.

Posted in: Health Insurance Reform

Related Questions

How can I find out if my hospital offers good care for my condition?

Where can I find information to compare nursing homes for quality?

Search HHS FAQs by questions or keywords:

Enter the terms you wish to search for.

Search
Content created by Digital Communications Division (DCD)
Content last reviewed April 20, 2023

ADDENDUM

Four key factors to follow along

- At 3 months pregnant I was having a pain in the left side of my groin. I went to Children's ER and was given instructions to "drink plenty of fluids. Eat a lot of vegetables & fruits" (10/21/96), 11:45a.m.. See: Discharge Instructions - Chapter 5
- Accused of having a "suspicions nature" and "having strong opinions regarding childbearing & medical care" (2/28/97), 12:45 p.m.. See: Patient Suspicions - Chapter 5
- Having an Epidural Anesthesia C-section whereas the Anesthesia never worked, before, during or after delivery (3/8/97), 12:15 p.m.. See: Operative Report - Chapter 10
- Being Discharged after the delivery with pre-eclampsia, High Blood Pressure of 180/105 including hyperreflexia without any BP medication (3/12/97). See: Discharge Summary - Chapter 16

AUTHOR'S BIO

Born and raised in Buffalo, NY, to Mr. Ulysese and Hazel Chillis, Author Eleanore Chillis, at the age of 3, moved into the newly built Ellicott Mall Housing Units. is where her love for community began. With her mother Hazel leaving her extended family, in Wrightsville, GA growing up in a close knit community was the family that was needed. Today, they meet annually, since 1999 at the well-attended Ellicott Mall Community Reunion in the nearby JFK Recreation Park.

Over a span of 22 years, her work experience involved some form of wellness and public service including Erie County Public Health, Environmental Health Services, Epidemiology Disease Control, Lead Poison Prevention, numerous Health (PODs) Point of Dispense and Retiring from Adult and Juvenile Probation. She has engaged in well over 250 community hours, earning countless certificates, certifications and awards. Her newest certification is in Fine Water Tasting from around the world, Tree Steward and Community Gardening.

Her previous work history entailed Buffalo City Hall Council District and City Tax Assessor's Offices; San Francisco, Hall of Justice Public Defenders, Mental Health Unit. And a formal background in Corporate Banking: Financial Planning and Control, Business Administration, Crocker National/Wells Fargo, San Francisco; Direct Response Marketing, Marine Midland/Hong Kong Shanghai, Buffalo.

Eleanore is the co-founder and COO of LifeSource Systems, Inc (LSS), a wellness 501c(3) not for profit organization that has spearheaded a successful pilot program to address African American woman health related obesity.

Currently, Eleanore's life's destiny and interest is to advocate for a Tribute Garden, Memorial Wall and Trail Walk in honor of mothers who have lost lives and or infants through childbirth. For families to reflect and communities to gather in memory of their loved one.

If you would like to share or possibly have your pregnancy story published in a storied related compilation, a future podcast discussion or simply provide the names of your loved one for the Tribute Garden aspirations,

Eleanore can be contacted on
(ladybugchillis@gmail.com)

INDEX

A

amniocentesis v, 23, 26, 88, 91, 103, 116, 117
amniotic fluid v, 9, 23, 79, 82, 88, 104, 116
anesthesia xxi, 7, 29, 51, 78, 79, 82, 97, 102, 106,
    108, 121, 122, 123, 147
anesthesiologist xxi, 47, 51, 97, 98, 123, 124, 125
anesthetic 106
autoimmune 85, 86, 104, 106

B

betamethasone 19, 23, 27, 28, 29, 81, 100, 104,
    106, 120
bladder blade 83
blood crossmatch 106
blood pressure v, vi, xx, 9, 19, 29, 62, 63, 72, 84, 87,
    106, 108, 109, 118, 147

C

caffeine 23, 106
catheter vi, 29, 47, 62, 63, 78, 81, 83, 106, 107,
    109, 128
cesarean scar 106, 107
complications xi, xx, 84, 85, 87, 92, 93, 106, 111, 118,
    131, 135, 144, 145
confirmed pregnancy due dates 106
contractions v, 23, 88, 106, 109, 118, 131
cornual angle fibroid 60, 83, 106
c-section 7, 51, 78, 79, 82, 99, 106, 108, 114, 115,
    119, 127, 147

D

deep tendon reflexes v, 89, 101, 103
deep vein thrombosis (DVT) v, 142
demerol 48, 63, 78, 79, 107
discharge 62, 72, 145, 146, 147
dorsal supine position 78, 107

E

eclampsia xx, 9, 19, 27, 29, 63, 78, 79, 84, 85, 101,
    103, 104, 107, 108, 118, 147
edema 10, 19, 107
embolism 86, 102, 142
epidural xxi, 7, 27, 29, 48, 51, 78, 79, 82, 124, 127,
    128, 147
estimated blood loss vi

F

fibroid 6, 10, 60, 61, 78, 79, 80, 83, 101, 106, 107,
    120, 121
findings xviii, xxi, 9, 60, 89

H

hemorrhage 28, 87, 88, 103, 107, 108, 109
hep catheter 29
hep prep vii, xxi
hip flexors xx, 9, 47, 54, 63, 71, 107
hyper-reflexes 63, 107
hypertension vi, vii, 9, 19, 29, 63, 79, 84, 106,
    107, 108

I

inter-uterine pregnancy 78, 79
intro-operative care plan & potential for anxiety
    xxi, 107
IUGR vi, 10, 78, 79

J

jagged bikini scar 107

K

kocher clamps 7, 82, 107

M

magnesium sulfate 5, 23, 27, 29, 52, 78, 81, 83, 101, 107, 109, 117, 118, 119
maternal iv, x, xii, xvii, xix, xx, xxi, 6, 7, 9, 88, 91, 92, 93, 94, 95, 96, 98, 99, 100, 101, 102, 103, 104, 105, 110, 111, 113, 114, 121
mayo scissors 82, 107
medical record xviii, xxi, 107, 130, 131, 142, 143
medical report viii, 78, 82, 130, 131
metzenbaum scissors 83, 107
morality iv, 107
morbidity iv, x, xii, xvii, xviii, xx, xxi, 73, 74, 85, 91, 99, 102, 104, 107, 110
morphine 48, 51
mortality iv, x, xii, xvii, xviii, xx, xxi, 7, 9, 28, 63, 73, 74, 85, 91, 92, 93, 94, 98, 99, 100, 102, 103, 104, 105, 107, 110, 111, 114, 121

O

oligohydramnios 78, 79, 80, 82, 88, 90, 91, 104
operation 108, 127, 132, 138
operative report xxi, 51, 78, 79, 82, 107, 147

P

pathology 90, 91, 107
placenta 83, 85, 87, 88, 90, 91, 99, 102, 103, 108, 119
planned pregnancy 2, 108
PNV prenatal vitamins 63
postoperative diagnosis 108
postpartum hemorrhage 87, 88, 103, 108, 109
preeclampsia 81, 84, 101, 102, 114, 118, 120
prenatal visits xxi, 6, 108
prenatal vitamins 63
preoperative 108
preoperative diagnosis 108
procedure xxi, 47, 48, 51, 60, 75, 79, 80, 82, 88, 102, 103, 107, 108, 109, 116, 121, 126, 127, 134, 135, 136, 137, 142, 143
ptsd 108
pulmonary blood clot 85, 86

R

recovery room vii, 51, 108

S

scalpel 47, 82, 108
sedation xxi, 48, 51, 78, 79, 82, 108
sedative 108
severe pre-eclampsia xx, 78, 79, 108
shock hemorrhage 108
SIDS vii, xviii, xxi, 73, 74

sonography 109
supine position 7, 47, 78, 82, 107, 109

T

tens xi, 109, 131
toradol 48, 78, 79, 109
toxemia 9, 109, 114
treatment iv, 6, 19, 28, 29, 53, 60, 61, 83, 84, 85, 87, 88, 97, 101, 102, 103, 109, 116, 120, 121, 125, 129, 130, 136, 142, 143, 144, 145
tubal ligation vii, 83, 109
tylenol 72

U

urinary catheter 109
uterine atony 109
uterine incision 78, 80, 83, 109

V

vesicouterine peritoneum 78, 83, 109

Printed in the United States
by Baker & Taylor Publisher Services